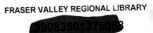
healthy mum,

happy baby

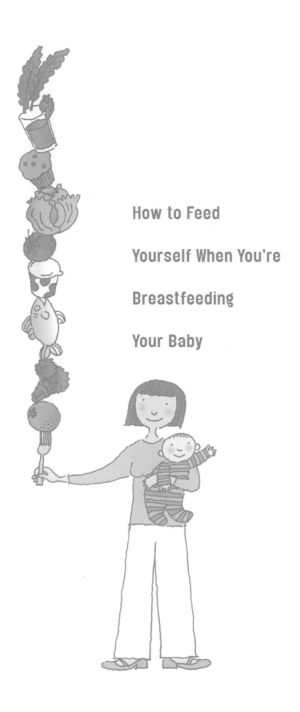

How to Feed

Yourself When You're

Breastfeeding

Your Baby

healthy mum, happy baby

ANNEMARIE TEMPELMAN-KLUIT

random house canada

Library and Archives Canada Cataloguing in Publication

Tempelman-Kluit, Annemarie
Healthy mum, happy baby : how to feed yourself when you're
breastfeeding your baby / Annemarie Tempelman-Kluit.

ISBN 978-0-679-31445-5

1. Breastfeeding.   2. Mothers—Nutrition.   3. Lactation—Nutritional
aspects.   4. Cookery.   I. Title.

RJ216.T44 2007   613.2'69   C2006-905697-8

Cover and text design: Kelly Hill

Illustrations: Joanne Vérroneau

Printed and bound in Canada

10 9 8 7 6 5 4 3 2 1

For Madeleine, who inspired this book,
and Lucy, who gestated along with it.

contents

INTRODUCTION

You thought you were prepared. You did all the prenatal things you were supposed to, from taking vitamins to practising yoga and taking birth classes. You read all the books, chose a theme for the nursery, and stocked up on an alarming amount of baby necessities from diapers to nasal aspirators. But as your due date drew near, you started to freak out about actually *having* this baby. Perfectly normal. Many mums, not surprisingly, fixate on the whole pain-of-childbirth thing, which can overshadow thoughts of the early days with your baby. But childbirth, as painful and protracted as it may be, doesn't last more than a day or two.

The early days of parenthood, on the other hand, threaten to never end. You're beyond exhaustion and you wonder if your baby—and consequently you—will ever sleep for more than two or three hours at a stretch. (Don't worry, you will!) And you worry. You worry that you haven't bonded with your baby, because despite what the books say, you can't seem to

1

distinguish between her different cries. You're sure that the contents of the diaper you're changing can't possibly be normal. You worry about your baby's growth and progress, compare her development to that of the other babies in your mums' group, and wonder how some other mothers seem to have time to apply mascara when you haven't even mastered the art of applying diaper cream.

And then there's breastfeeding, which brings a whole different set of worries and challenges. Why is it that something that's supposed to be so natural doesn't necessarily come so naturally? Do you have enough milk or too much? Does your baby nurse too frequently or not frequently enough? My first daughter refused point-blank to nurse. She'd shriek angrily at the merest whiff of a nipple, as though I were offering poison rather than breast milk. "I've never seen anything like this," announced the mystified lactation consultant I visited. But I was determined to breastfeed. Breast milk was, after all, best. All the experts recommended exclusive breastfeeding for six months, and my milk was brimming with long-term health benefits for my baby (and don't think thoughts of increased weight loss hadn't entered my mind). So, I rented an electric breast pump and spent many hours boiling bits of pumping paraphernalia while the rest of my household slumbered. We fed my daughter my milk with spoons, syringes, cups, and finally, despite my fears of nipple confusion, bottles. Mysteriously, when she was three and a half weeks old she took the breast and never looked back.

My trials and tribulations meant I amassed quite the extensive breastfeeding library. In one book by the well-known Dr. William Sears, I discovered a list of nutrient-dense, more

2

bang-for-your-buck foods for breastfeeding mothers. Despite all my reading and preparation for motherhood, it wasn't until I came across this list that I twigged to the fact I was still eating for two. I knew that what I ate would flavour my breast milk, and that I needed to stay well hydrated and eat more than I had pre-pregnancy, but I'd never really considered how much my diet would affect my baby's growth and development or my health and energy. Great. Now I had something else to worry about. Was my baby getting enough of the vitamins she needed? Would her IQ be forever affected if I didn't eat enough fish or flaxseeds? If I existed solely on fast food would my breast milk still be better for my baby than formula? And how exactly did I go about feeding myself so I could feed her better?

Most books I'd read recommended that a nursing mother continue to eat as healthily as she had done while she was pregnant. Easier said than done. In those early, hazy days of new parenthood, we were subsisting on freezer meals, takeout, and dinners my mother brought over. Not a recipe for long-term success (but awfully nice while it lasted). What I needed was more than just advice on the kinds of foods I should be eating. I needed some sort of sense of how exactly a new mum can still manage to eat healthily while caring for a newborn. How do you carve out time to cook and eat when you don't even have time to empty the dishwasher? There didn't seem to be anything out there to help me figure all of this out. And my need was increasingly desperate. Rifling through the kitchen cupboards at three in the morning trying to find something to eat that wasn't toast or chocolate seemed crazy. My husband and my two-month-old daughter were both sound asleep, but my desperate need for food was outweighing even my desperate

3

need for sleep. I just wanted something, anything, healthy to fill the enormous and permanent hole that seemed to have taken up the space recently vacated by my baby. As I wolfed down yet another bowl of cold cereal, I wished my prenatal classes had covered eating with a newborn and stressed more firmly the importance of stocking your freezer with more than a few frozen meals. I wished I'd had some inkling of how hungry I'd be, how my diet would affect my energy and my breast milk, how eating well would help with the transition into motherhood, and, quite frankly, how much help I'd need. I realized I really needed a guide to stocking my pantry with handy snack foods and ingredients for quick meals. I needed a set of healthy recipes that would be fast to make and easy to double and store in the freezer. I needed reliable, uncomplicated, up-to-date nutritional information. I needed to know that if ever there was a time to ask for help and to be specific in what I needed—like washing the dishes or cleaning the bathroom or bringing over dinner—this was it. And I needed to know that sometimes, no matter how good my intentions and how well stocked my pantry, there would be circumstances that would call for a guilt-free chocolate bar, a big bowl of chips, or a glass of wine. And if I needed this, surely other mums did too.

I started to poll my new-mum friends. Had they heard of this list of foods that were considered optimal for breastfeeding? Were they following any dietary recommendations? New mums today are overwhelmed with the pressure to give their babies every advantage from breast milk to organic-cotton onesies to infant flash cards. Worrying that they too were missing some crucial piece of the mummy puzzle, my friends jumped onto the worry wagon with me. Would I e-mail them the list?

4

What else should they be eating? I began to interview dietitians and lactation consultants. I became a regular on the Health Canada and American Academy of Pediatrics websites. I also became the go-to girl for my friends and their friends with breastfeeding questions, and in turn they shared with me their tips and tricks for making life with a newborn easier. Slowly my idea for *Healthy Mum, Happy Baby* grew; it would be a cookbook for breastfeeding mums, but would also focus on helping make their lives just a little easier.

All the recipes in *Healthy Mum, Happy Baby* have been tested by real mums with real babies wailing, cooing, or even sleeping in the background. Most of the snacks are designed for one-handed eating to free up the other for breastfeeding, stroller pushing, or playing. The chapter on stocking your pantry is designed to help you fill up your cupboards pre-baby, to help you make better food choices. I've also provided a chapter on the basics of a healthy breastfeeding diet.

And while organic-cotton onesies and infant flash cards may have their place in your baby's life, don't forget that what your baby really wants more than anything is you. I truly hope that the advice collected between these pages helps you worry a little less, keeps your new-mum guilt simmering instead of boiling over, reminds you to trust your instincts more than the experts who've never met your baby, and eat a little better so you have more energy for yourself and for your baby. Enjoy.

5

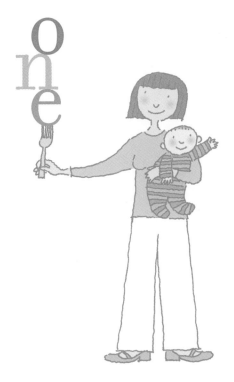

one

EATING FOR TWO

1

BREASTFEEDING: AS GOOD AS IT GETS

You may be surprised as a new mum by how much work breastfeeding can be. If your pregnancy didn't convince you that you're no longer in charge at your house, breastfeeding certainly will. After all, when it comes to eating, that little person you're feeding calls the shots.

That lesson was brought doubly home to me after the birth of my second daughter, Lucy. I had figured that after all the problems and stress we'd had getting Madeleine to breastfeed that I'd paid my dues and done my time, but no. Lucy was more eager to sleep than nurse, and once we'd managed to wake her, a feat in itself involving ice packs and near-nakedness in January, she'd feed quite literally for an hour on end. Her latch seemed perfect, my milk supply seemed fine, and I didn't appear to have thrush, yet I developed agonizingly sore, crying-when-she-latched nipples. Once again I read books and consulted experts, but no one could pinpoint the problem, which luckily resolved itself when Lucy was almost two months old.

9

Breastfeeding can be surprising on many levels. One yoga-teaching, earth-mother type I know who just assumed breastfeeding would be a blissful experience was taken aback to find it tedious and frustrating. Other women who expect it to be a chore are surprised by how much they enjoy it. If you are finding breastfeeding tedious, it may help to remind yourself that you're giving your baby the very best—your milk— and to consider each feeding an opportunity to be more in the moment and more patient. It may also help to position

Taking Good Care of "The Girls"

Your extra-bodacious tatas are probably getting a lot more attention than ever before. But instead of lift and perkiness, you're now worrying about problems like leaking, cracking, bleeding, and blocking up. Sigh. Your breasts are now yet another thing that needs your tender loving care. Here are a few tips on how to keep them as healthy as possible:

- Air dry them after feedings.
- Avoid washing them with soap.
- Express a few drops of breast milk and rub them into your nipples after each feeding.
- Avoid using any creams on your nipples, except pure lanolin, unless recommended or prescribed by your health care professional.
- Use 100 percent cotton breast pads, or disposable breast pads without plastic lining, so your nipples can breath.

your nursing chair near the television and indulge in some tube time while you nurse. I've known mothers who worked with their babies to time feedings around their favourite shows.

Sometimes breastfeeding can seem overwhelming and there will be times when you wonder why you ever thought it was a good idea in the first place. The following primer is designed to help get you through those moments.

BREASTFEEDING . . . Is Best for Babies Because

- Your breast milk is perfectly in tune with your baby. The proteins, fats, and minerals in your milk adjust according to the time of day, the seasons, and your baby's changing needs.
- The antibodies in your milk reduce the rate of infection for your baby and increase her protection against ear, respiratory, and gastrointestinal infections.
- Breast milk increases protection against illnesses such as childhood diabetes.
- Breast milk increases protection against allergies.
- Breast milk may help cognitive development.

. . . Is Best for Mothers Because

- Breastfeeding releases hormones that help the uterus contract after birth.
- Breastfeeding helps protect against breast and ovarian cancers.
- Breastfeeding helps with postpartum weight loss.
- Breastfeeding helps prevent osteoporosis.

11

... Makes Life Easier Because

- Although it may not always seem easier when you're the only one who can feed your baby, breast milk is always fresh and ready to serve.
- Breastfeeding saves time; there's no sterilizing, mixing, or washing of bottles involved.
- Breastfeeding saves money; despite a mother's increased caloric intake, it still costs far less to feed you than to keep your baby in formula, bottles, and nipples.

Health Canada, the Canadian Paediatric Society, and the American Academy of Pediatrics are now all in line with the World Health Organization's 2001 recommendation that an infant should be exclusively breastfed for six months. Exclusive breastfeeding means your baby gets only breast milk (including expressed breast milk), as well as vitamin D supplements and any medications he may need. While this is ideal, any breast milk is better than no breast milk, and for various reasons it may be necessary to supplement with formula, wean earlier than planned, or start solids before six months for your baby's health. There are also some situations where breastfeeding may not be recommended.

When Breast May Not Be Best

The following medical conditions may prevent you from breastfeeding, but your decision should be made in tandem with your health care professional.

HIV/AIDS It's not recommended that HIV antibody–positive

mothers breastfeed as there's a risk of transmitting the virus to their babies.

Tuberculosis Though rarely transmitted in breast milk, tuberculosis (TB) can be transmitted by exposure to sputum, and so mothers with active TB should only breastfeed if they are receiving appropriate therapy and are not considered infectious.

Preventing Blocked Milk Ducts

Blocked ducts are caused by inadequate drainage of milk, and if untreated, can lead to mastitis, which you definitely don't want. If you find a firm lump in your breast that hurts when you touch it, chances are you have a blocked milk duct. The initial treatment is to continue nursing. You'll know your blocked duct has become mastisized if, in addition to a hard, swollen lump you have a fever and flu-like symptoms. Here are some tips on avoiding blocked ducts:

• Wear a nursing bra, preferably without underwire. If you are wearing a nursing bra with underwire make sure you have it fitted by a professional.

• If you are wearing a regular bra, flip it under, not over, your breasts while breastfeeding.

• Experiment with different feeding positions to ensure all your ducts get drained.

• Let your baby fully finish one breast before switching.

• If you do feel a lump, massage the blocked area in the direction of your nipple while in the shower or while nursing.

13

Hepatitis B If you acquire Hepatitis B while breastfeeding, it's important that your baby be immunized against it as soon as possible.

Herpes Unless you actually have lesions on or around your nipples, the virus is unlikely to make it into your breast milk.

Breast milk may be best, but feeling guilty because you can't breastfeed, or breastfeed for as long as you'd like, isn't beneficial to you or your baby. Your experiences with breastfeeding, like parenting, will teach you that things don't always go by the book, and that patience, flexibility, and pragmatism will take you far. As will basing your breastfeeding decisions on fact and not fiction. Let's clear up some popular misconceptions.

Breastfeeding Myths Debunked

1. BREASTFEEDING TIES YOU DOWN.

Not necessarily. While breastfeeding is definitely a time commitment, it shouldn't prevent you from ever leaving the house. As long as you are comfortable nursing in public, babies are happy to be out and about exploring the world. And not having to drag bottles and formula around means you can travel relatively lightly. You'll be amazed how many people don't mind if you show up with your tot in tow. I took my bottle-resistant 3-month-old to the dentist with me where she sat happily in a bouncy chair beside the receptionist being admired by all.

Initially, breastfeeding in public may seem a bit daunting, so take a friend along for moral support, or meet another

14

breastfeeding mother and do it together. Once you've prac-tised a few times, you'll feel more comfortable with the whole process.

If you need to get out on your own for a while and your baby takes a bottle, you can leave expressed breast milk for your partner or caregiver to feed your baby while you're out. Although a breastfed baby who won't take a bottle may make you long for the days of the wet nurse, you can still pop out on your own for an hour or two between feedings.

2. BREASTFEEDING WILL MAKE MY BREASTS SAG.

You won't realize just how elastic your breasts are until your tiny tot starts tugging on them. Genetics and body type are the factors that determine how perky they'll stay, not breastfeed-ing. You can help the situation further by wearing supportive bras and working your pectoral muscles.

3. A BREASTFEEDING MOTHER HAS TO DRINK MILK TO MAKE MILK.

Milk doesn't produce milk. A diet full of vegetables, fruits, grains, and proteins provides all that's necessary to produce milk.

4. MY BABY'S ALWAYS HUNGRY, I MUST NOT HAVE ENOUGH MILK.

Breast milk digests more easily than formula, so breastfed babies may eat more frequently than formula-fed babies. But every baby eats differently—a fact you'll be able to attest to if you've had more than one. Some are frequent nibblers, others feed longer and less often. The best way to ensure a plentiful milk supply is to feed your baby when he's hungry and not limit the length of feedings.

15

5. RICE CEREAL WILL HELP MY BABY SLEEP THROUGH THE NIGHT.

If only it were that simple. Well-meaning friends and relatives will often suggest you start solids sooner than you'd planned to help you and your baby sleep longer at night. There are many theories and philosophies about babies and sleep, and no two are the same, however almost every expert agrees that rice cereal will not help your baby sleep longer.

Ideally, babies should be exclusively breastfed for the first six months, but some mothers find it necessary to introduce solids earlier. You should try to wait until at least four months to introduce solids, but after that, if you feel your baby needs more, consult your doctor.

6. BREASTFEEDING PREVENTS PREGNANCY.

Believe this one and you may be welcoming another little one ten months from now. Breastfeeding *may* be up to 98 percent effective as a birth control method if your baby receives nothing but breast milk on demand—meaning no solids, no pacifiers, and no formula. But why take the risk if you're not ready to conceive again? Talk to your doctor about the most effective form of birth control for your lifestyle.

16

2

THE BUILDING BLOCKS OF
A BREASTFEEDING DIET

I couldn't believe how hungry I was when I started breastfeeding. Eating for two had been one of my favourite parts of pregnancy (once I got past my nauseating first trimester) and almost made up for my swelling girth and continual need to pee. In contrast, when I started to breast-feed, eating for two became a chore, a trial, a bodily necessity that I couldn't seem to satisfy. I'd known that the early days of parenthood would be exhausting, but I hadn't expected that for me, hunger would more often than not trump tiredness. Gone were the days of eating mindfully and savouring the taste of food; instead I discovered I could cram an entire muffin into my mouth, that yogurt was just as good eaten straight from the container, and that I could eat cheese and crackers, talk on the phone, and rock a fussy baby all at the same time. It wasn't until a Sunday dinner with my extended family that I realized how far I'd fallen. As I sat at the laden table, I felt as if I hadn't eaten in months. I couldn't wait for everyone to be seated—a two-minute delay felt like two hours stretched ahead of me. By the time everyone had sat down at the table, my plate and mouth were full. I stopped chewing only long enough to mumble through my food, "Sorry Mum, I couldn't wait, but this is really good!"

In retrospect, it's not surprising I was so hungry. Your body needs an extra 500 calories or so a day to make the 23 to 27 ounces of breast milk your baby needs each day. Though not all women experience the kind of intense hunger I did, your nutritional needs do increase when you're breastfeeding. With a few important exceptions that I'll cover later in this chapter, the quality of your diet will not hugely impact the quality of your breast milk. If you don't get enough nutrients, your body puts your baby first and depletes your store of vitamins and minerals to make sure that baby gets hers. However an inadequate diet can affect the quantity of milk you produce and the quality of your health now and into the future. If you don't get enough nutrients, you could experience vitamin and mineral deficiencies that could affect your health later on in life. Eating a good diet during your early days as a parent will also give you the energy you need to meet the enormous demands being made on your stamina and strength, and replaces nutrients lost during pregnancy, like calcium, vitamin D, iron, and folic acid. A healthy diet also ensures you get the nutrients your baby can only get from you, such as essential fats. And eating enough fibre and drinking plenty of fluids will help keep you regular—a huge concern for all mums in the early days after birth, and even more so for those who've had C-sections. In modern mothering there's a tendency to think

Working in Some Working Out

Exercise helps with postpartum weight loss, boosts your mood and energy, and can help firm those jiggly bits that grew along with your baby. But it can be difficult to work a regular fitness class into your breastfeeding and baby-care schedule, especially if you don't have a babysitter. Here are some suggestions for how you might slot in some exercise time:

- Look for local community centres that offer childcare during fitness classes.
- Join a strollercise, mum-and-baby workout, or mum-and-baby Pilates class, which are becoming more common at community centres and gyms.
- Check to see if your prenatal yoga studio offers or can recommend a postnatal yoga class, or a mum-and-babe class.
- Explore your neighbourhood with your baby in a carrier or stroller for ten to twenty minutes a day, or walk to your mums's group with other local, like-minded mums.

If you can't manage to fit in any formal exercise, it's important to remember that the only person who thinks that pushing a baby up a hill in a stroller laden with groceries isn't exercise is someone who hasn't tried it.

20

that becoming a mother means always putting your child's needs above your own, but taking care of yourself and eating well will help you become the mother you want to be. Not necessarily the mother with the mascara on but the mother with energy to interact with her baby, and the one who sets a great example for her child and family about how and what to eat.

As a new mum it's natural to be more than a little obsessed with losing your baby weight. Ubiquitous news stories and photos of celebrity mothers who effortlessly shrink back to their pre-baby stick figures create unrealistic expectations. But let's get real: it took more than nine months to put on the baby weight, and for those of us without a chef and personal trainer, it's probably going to take at least that long to take it off.

The first six weeks of breastfeeding is definitely not a time to diet because your milk supply is still being established. After that, if you're losing more than a pound a week, your rapid weight loss may result in the release of toxins from your body fat into your milk. So if you're losing more than a pound a week, you're probably not eating enough.

Luckily, breastfeeding releases hormones that help your uterus return to its pre-pregnancy size and shape, and studies have shown that mums who breastfeed tend to lose more weight than mums who don't. But every body reacts differently; some women lose pounds steadily and return to their regular weight while still breastfeeding, while others stubbornly hold onto the extra weight until their baby starts eating solids. No matter how eager you might be to shed the extra pounds, you must be patient and careful. Give your body time to recover and don't ignore your feelings of hunger. And don't start diets that require you to eliminate or drastically reduce one type of food, such as carbohydrates or fat—not enough is known about how these restrictive diets affect your breast milk. You're already counting wet and dirty diapers and the number of times your baby feeds in a day, so the last thing you need to add into the mix is counting calories. Instead, trust your body's cues and eat if you're hungry, drink enough to keep your thirst at bay, and aim for regular, well-balanced meals and snacks. Focus on foods that pack a nutrient wallop to keep you and your baby well fuelled, and don't let the occasional bowl of ice cream or stop at the drive-through throw you off course.

The best way to ensure you get a healthy, well-balanced diet is to eat regular meals and snacks from each of the four food groups in Canada's Food Guide to Healthy Eating (see Health Canada's website at www.hc-sc.gc.ca). These are grain products, vegetables and fruit, milk products, and meat and alternatives.

> ## Dehydrated?
>
> Fatigue is one of the first signs of dehydration, so despite the fact you won't be sure if you're feeling fatigued because you haven't slept much for two months or you simply haven't had enough to drink, downing an extra glass of water won't hurt.

GRAIN PRODUCTS
Recommended servings a day: 5 to 12
A serving is: 1 slice of bread
                   ½ of a bagel
                   ¾ cup of cold cereal

$^3/_4$ cup of hot cereal

$^1/_2$ cup of cooked rice

$^1/_2$ cup of cooked pasta

With grains, it's always best to choose whole-grain products like whole wheat bread and brown rice rather than refined grains like white bread and white rice. Whole grains contain all three parts of the grain including the bran, the germ, and the kernel or endosperm. Bran is a good source of fibre and contains B vitamins and antioxidants. The germ is where all the really good stuff is concentrated. It's packed with nutrients such as niacin, thiamin, riboflavin, vitamin E, magnesium, phosphorus, iron, and zinc, and contains most of the grain's protein. Neither the bran nor the germ are present in refined grains; all that's left is the endosperm, which contains lots of carbohydrates and some protein but few nutrients. Whole grains add fibre to your diet and can also help lower your risk for heart disease, cancer, and diabetes. So try adding more whole grains to your diet whenever you can.

Upping the Ante: Many of the recipes in this book include whole grains where possible, but here are some further suggestions for how you might add more whole grains to your diet:

- Start the day off with a bowl of large-flake oatmeal or high-fibre cold cereal rather than cornflakes or instant oatmeal.
- Buy whole-grain bread, tortillas, and pasta.
- Instead of cooking white rice, experiment with brown rice, barley, bulgur, or quinoa.

23

- In recipes calling for all-purpose flour, try replacing half with whole wheat flour.
- In recipes calling for dry breadcrumbs, try replacing them with rolled oats or crushed bran cereal.

VEGETABLES AND FRUIT

Recommended servings a day: 5 to 10

A serving is: ½ cup of cooked vegetables

1 cup of leafy greens

1 medium piece of fruit such as an apple or orange

¼ cup dried fruit

We all know that vegetables and fruit are good for us. They're chock full of vitamins, minerals, and fibre, and they're naturally low in sodium and calories. They also contain phytochemicals, which are compounds that may reduce the risk of heart disease, diabetes, and some cancers. Many vegetables and fruits are also good sources of antioxidants, which slow cell and tissue damage. But don't limit yourself to just apples and broccoli all the time; be sure to eat as wide a variety as you can. Kiwis are high in vitamin C, while bananas are full of potassium. Asparagus is high in folate, while carrots are good sources of vitamin A. Eating a wide array of vegetables and fruit, especially orange, dark green, and other dark-coloured varieties, will ensure you get the wide range of vitamins and minerals you need. Eating produce that's in season is a good way to expand your repertoire. And the produce will be fresher, better tasting, and lower priced to boot. A visit to your local farmer's market with your baby is both an opportunity to stock up from local suppliers and a chance to introduce your baby to the fact that food doesn't originate at the grocery store.

Frozen and canned vegetables and fruit are also excellent sources of nutrition. They're usually packaged immediately after being picked and consequently often contain more nutrients than produce that has been shipped long distances. Be aware that canned vegetables can contain high amounts of sodium, so try to choose those without added salt. Choose canned fruit that has been packed in water or fruit juice rather than syrup—who needs the extra sugar?

Upping the Ante: Trying to get 5 to 10 servings of vegetables and fruit a day can be challenging even when you're well rested and rational, never mind sleep deprived and hormonal. Here are some simple tips to help you reach your recommended intake:

- Start the day off with a Basic Berry Smoothie (see recipe on page 86).
- Top your breakfast cereal or oatmeal with fruit such as sliced bananas, fresh or frozen berries, or applesauce.
- Expand upon a basic omelette by adding lots of chopped veggies such as onions, tomatoes, bell peppers, mushrooms, spinach, and asparagus. Cooked vegetables left over from last night's dinner, such as potatoes, carrots, and green beans, can also be tossed in.
- Have a bowl of vegetable soup for lunch or as an appetizer for dinner. Hot vegetable soups such as minestrone are wonderful in winter, while cold soups like gazpacho are refreshing in summer.

25

- When making a sandwich, try to include at least three vegetables, such as lettuce, tomatoes, cucumbers, avocado and bell peppers.
- When making tuna or egg salad, try adding some chopped onion, celery, bell peppers, or grated carrot.
- Eat dips with carrots, celery, broccoli, cauliflower, and bell peppers.
- Unpeeled, unwashed carrots may cost less but if you'll eat more veggies by buying those handy bags of ready-to-eat baby carrots then they're worth it.
- Give yourself an extra serving of vegetables with your dinner.
- When making stew, pasta sauce, or chili, add a few extra carrots, some more chopped bell peppers, or another handful of mushrooms.
- Try topping your tacos, burritos, or quesadillas with lots of lettuce and chopped tomatoes, bell peppers, and avocado.
- When ordering pizza, ask for lots of vegetable toppings and half the amount of cheese.

DAIRY

Recommended servings a day: 3 to 4

A serving is: 8 oz of milk

$^3/_4$ cup of yogurt

2 oz (the size of 3 dominos) of cheese

Dairy is a key source of calcium, which is essential for strong teeth and bones. If you don't get enough calcium in your diet, you could be at increased risk for developing osteoporosis later

26

in life. Calcium also helps your muscles and nervous system function properly, and helps regulate blood pressure.

In addition to calcium, dairy products provide protein, B vitamins, and minerals such as selenium, zinc, phosphorous, potassium, and magnesium. Most milk is fortified with vitamin D, which helps our bodies absorb calcium. Cultured milk products like yogurt or buttermilk may contain probiotics, or good bacteria, which can help maintain a healthy intestinal tract and help prevent some illnesses.

Because many dairy products are high in saturated fat, which is the principle dietary cause of heart disease, it's important to choose low- or non-fat dairy products such as skim milk, non-fat yogurt, and low-fat cheese and sour cream.

When You Can't Do Dairy: Not everyone can or likes to drink milk, so if you're one of those people, how do you get all the calcium you need? Because it's harder to absorb the mineral from supplements than dietary sources, it's best to get your calcium from food. Good non-dairy dietary sources of calcium include canned sardines and salmon with the bones; calcium-fortified orange juice and soy milk; sesame seeds; almonds; dark green leafy vegetables such as collard greens, spinach, kale, and bok choy; and cooked oysters and scallops.

MEAT AND ALTERNATIVES
Recommended servings a day: 2 to 3

A serving is:	2–3 ounces (the size of a deck of cards) of beef, poultry, or fish
	1 egg
	$^{1}/_{3}$ cup of beans

27

⅓ cup of lentils

⅓ cup of firm tofu

2 tbsp peanut butter

Meat and alternatives provide us with B vitamins, iron, zinc, and, above all, protein. Protein is one of the body's essential building blocks, and we need it for the growth and repair of tissues. Because it's rare for a North American to be deficient in protein, you probably don't need to worry about getting enough. But you should consider what types of protein-rich foods you include in your diet.

Meat and poultry, excellent sources of high-quality protein, also contain cholesterol and saturated fat. You can reduce this fat by trimming meat and removing the skin from poultry. Fish, which is also high in protein, is low in cholesterol and saturated fat. Nuts and seeds are an excellent source of plant protein, and they're packed with nutrients and are cholesterol free. However, because nuts are high in fat and calories, it's a good idea to limit how many you eat. Legumes— beans, peas, and lentils—are high in protein, folate, potassium, iron, and magnesium and are low in fat with no cholesterol. Legumes are also a good source of fibre and contain phytochemicals, which may help prevent chronic diseases such as cardiovascular disease and some cancers. All these are convincing reasons to try to eat less meat and more fish and legumes.

Upping the Ante: To increase your intake of legumes, try the following:

- Eat soups that contain legumes, such as minestrone, pasta e fagioli, black bean, lentil, and split pea.
- Add chickpeas, kidney beans, and lentils to your salads.
- Snack on dips made of legumes, like hummus and black bean dip. You can also use hummus as a sandwich spread or use it in a pita with tomatoes, cucumbers, and lettuce.
- Replace half the meat in a taco, stir-fry, stew, or casserole with beans.

The following recipes will help you get protein from a combination of animal and legume sources:

Chicken and Black Bean Quesadillas (page 138)
Chicken, Bean, and Spinach Soup (page 140)
Pollo Salsa Verde (page 142)
White Chili (page 144)

The four major food groups are the building blocks of a well balanced diet for everyone. But breastfeeding makes special demands on your body and some nutrients are particularly important for you and your baby.

Necessary Nutrients

The nutrients breastfeeding women are most likely to be deficient in are essential fats, folic acid, and vitamin D. Here's the lowdown on these crucial components of a healthy breastfeeding diet.

THE FATS OF LIFE

Though, in general, your diet has little effect on the quality of your breast milk, there is one glaring, important exception: fat. The type of fat you consume directly correlates to the type of fat in your breast milk. Fats provide energy, carry fat-soluble vitamins from our food into our bodies, help us feel full, and help to keep our skin and hair healthy. On the flip side, fat has double the concentration of calories found in protein and carbohydrates. And not all fat is created equal. "Bad" fats raise your cholesterol, which increases your risk for heart disease and stroke, while "good" fats can reduce cholesterol levels, help protect against stroke, and support the immune system. Then there are essential fatty acids, or EFAs, which are critical for your baby's brain and visual development.

Saturated and trans fats, which tend to be solid at room temperature, are both "bad" fats, although trans fats could be considered even worse. Saturated fats are found in red meat and full-fat dairy products and they raise your cholesterol level. Trans fats, which are often found in processed baked goods and fried foods, not only raise your bad cholesterol, or LDL, but they also lower your good cholesterol, or HDL, which protects against heart attack and stroke and supports your immune system. In terms of breast milk, trans fats also reduce the overall levels of fat in breast milk and inhibit the absorption of EFAs. Canada's new food labelling laws require companies to list saturated and trans fats on their nutrition labels, so it's easier to watch out for and avoid them.

Monounsaturated and polyunsaturated fats, which tend to be liquid at room temperature, are "good" fats and they both reduce bad cholesterol. Monounsaturated fats are found in olive, canola, and peanut oils; nuts; seeds; and avocados, while polyunsaturated fats are found in vegetable oils; nuts; seeds; and fatty fish. Then there are the very, very good fats, the EFAs. Omega-3 fatty acids, which include alpha-linoleic acid (ALA), eicosapentaenoic acid (EPA) and docosahexaenoic acid (DHA) are all EFAs. The body coverts ALA into EPA, which fights infections, and DHA, which is necessary for brain and visual development and function. Because our bodies do not produce EFAs we can get them only from food, and the two main sources of omega-3s are fatty, cold-water fish and flaxseeds. Recent research shows that the conversion of ALA from plant sources such as flaxseeds to EPA and DHA is low, so fish is really the best source of omega-3. I guess our mothers were right, fish truly is brain food.

Fish Facts: With the negative press that's been circulating about fish recently, there's lots of confusion about whether fish is a truly healthy food or is loaded with mercury and other toxins and therefore best avoided.

Fish is high in protein, low in saturated fat, and one of the best sources of omega-3 fatty acids around. Unfortunately some fish is high in mercury, which can be harmful to developing fetuses, breastfed infants, and young children—and it's not great for grown-ups either. Farmed salmon, we now hear, contains cancer-causing dioxins. So are we better off to stick with flaxseed oil and omega-3 eggs and never eat fish again? Hardly—we just need to be aware of the *type* of fish we're eating.

Long-lived, larger fish that feed on other fish accumulate the highest levels of mercury and should therefore be avoided altogether by pregnant and breastfeeding women, and young

31

children. These types of fish include tuna steaks, swordfish, shark, marlin or tilefish, king mackerel, muskellunge, and walleye. "White," "albacore," or "bluefin" canned tuna should be enjoyed no more than once a month, as should bluefish, grouper, orange roughy, and lobster. However, canned "light" tuna, usually skipjack, yellowfin, or tongol, is smaller and shorter-lived than albacore tuna, and therefore contains less mercury. Fatty, short-lived wild fish such as sardines, salmon, and sablefish are the most beneficial and the safest species. As well, feel free to enjoy anchovies, bass, clams, cod, crab, flounder, haddock, halibut, herring, mackerel (but not king mackerel), oysters, perch, pollock, scallops, shrimp, skate, snapper, sole, squid, tilapia, and trout regularly.

That still leaves the question of salmon. Farmed salmon generally has higher levels of dioxins than wild because of the type of feed the fish is given. So you may want to stick to wild salmon. However, be aware that dioxin levels in farmed salmon still fall within government guidelines, and that you can cut down on them by removing the skin and the brown fat before cooking, and allowing the fat to drain away during cooking. Canned salmon is almost always wild salmon, and smart producers usually indicate that on the label.

Popping fish oil capsules might seem to be the easiest way to get all your omega-3s, but, like any supplement, fish oil capsules don't have the nutrition of the whole food, and it's unknown whether the other nutrients in the whole food may work with the omega fat to provide the health benefits. Unlike the fish, the supplements don't contain vitamin D. Fish liver oils have potentially high levels of vitamin A and may be contaminated with mercury or other pollutants. Do your research to ensure you're getting a "pure" version if you do want to take supplements.

So don't cut out salmon and other fish from your diet. Get thee to a fishmonger and make informed choices. The vitamins and EFAs are just too beneficial to pass up.

Upping the Ante: Here are some suggestions for ensuring you get some EFAs every day:

- Eat fresh, frozen, or canned fatty fish such as salmon, anchovies, sardines, and mackerel two to three times a week.
- Use ground flaxseeds in baking; on top of cereal, cottage cheese, and salad; or in smoothies. The ground seeds are a better source of EFAs than whole seeds or oil, though they're good too. Ground flaxseeds can be stored in an opaque, airtight container in the fridge for up to three months or whole flaxseeds can be ground fresh in a coffee grinder as needed.
- Make nuts and seeds part of your daily snacks.
- Look for omega-3-enriched products when you're shopping. Omega-3 eggs, for example, contain eight to ten times more omega-3s than regular eggs.

The following recipes will help you get your share of omega-3s from fish sources:

Open-Face Sardine Sandwiches (page 112)
Salmon au Poivre (page 124)
Salmon with Citrus Yogurt Sauce (page 126)

33

Broccoli and Anchovy Orecchiette (page 128)

Salmon and Spinach Quiche (page 154)

FOLIC ACID

Folic acid, or vitamin B9, helps form hemoglobin in red blood cells and build new cells. It is the only vitamin routinely lacking in women's diets in Western countries. The best sources of folic acid are green vegetables, cabbage, orange juice, and beans. But it's not easy for women to get their recommended daily dose of 400 micrograms of folic acid from diet alone. Thus all women of child-bearing age are advised to take a daily supplement. Folic acid is vital to the development of a baby's nervous system, and therefore key in preventing neural tube defects. It also ensures a baby's continued normal development. Because breastfeeding mums don't have much folic acid stored in their bodies—most folic acid is excreted in urine—they should take a daily supplement of 400 micrograms. If it's hard to find that specific dosage, you may need to get yours from a multivitamin. Be sure to discuss this with your health care provider.

VITAMIN D

Vitamin D is necessary for absorbing calcium into your bones. Dietary sources include fatty fish, egg yolks, and fortified milk and yogurt. (Sadly, cheese and ice cream are not vitamin D fortified.) Vitamin D is also naturally produced in our bodies by exposure to sunlight. But many Canadian climes are less than sunny, and dermatologists suggest restricting sun exposure to reduce your chances of developing skin cancer. Because of this, your baby is unlikely to get much sun exposure. Breast milk doesn't contain a lot of vitamin D, so Health Canada, in tandem with the Dietitians of Canada and the Canadian Paediatric Society, recommends that all breastfed infants take a daily vitamin D supplement from birth until they're a year old or are receiving adequate vitamin D from other sources. Vitamin D is very important for mothers' health too, and they are advised to get their supply from food sources.

TO SUPPLEMENT OR NOT TO SUPPLEMENT

As long as you are eating a healthy, nutritious diet, you probably needn't take any supplements except for 400 micrograms of folic acid a day. But it's best to discuss your specific needs and circumstances with your health care professional.

Feel free to finish any leftover prenatal vitamins once your baby's born, but after that be aware that most prenatal vitamins have more iron than a postnatal mother needs, and getting too much iron can be harmful.

In addition to getting these building blocks of a healthy breastfeeding diet, be sure to drink plenty of liquids each day. Most mums notice that they become much thirstier when they start breastfeeding. An easy way to stay on top of your thirst is to have a glass of water each time you nurse.

3

EAT, DRINK, BUT BE WARY

From the moment your pregnancy becomes public knowledge you're bombarded with advice. Everyone from your mother to perfect strangers has an opinion on everything from diapers to sleeping arrangements to what you should eat and avoid while pregnant and breastfeeding. More than just overwhelming, this unsolicited advice, no matter how well meaning, can leave you confused and worried that you might be causing your baby irreparable harm. Can you indulge your vices a little and have a glass of wine with dinner now you're breastfeeding? Must you avoid all caffeine, including (please, God, no) chocolate? Will spicy foods give your baby colic? Are there toxins in your breast milk? If you eat peanuts will your baby develop a peanut allergy? Once you've got the whole grains and essential fats info down, you need the answers to these important questions and more.

37

ALCOHOL

Basically, almost everything that goes into your body gets into your breast milk. Alcohol appears in breast milk in the same concentration as it does in your bloodstream, and heavy alcohol consumption can mess with your milk supply, your baby, and your mothering in general. However, this does not mean you can't drink at all. An occasional, well-timed glass of wine or beer isn't frowned upon and can help a new mum relax a little.

After nine-plus months of being the designated driver, I was hoping to celebrate my first child's birth with a glass of champagne. Thoughts of celebrating fell by the wayside when Madeleine refused to nurse. Was it my milk or lack thereof? Was it inexperience? Perhaps there was some mysterious misalignment between her mouth and my nipples? After three days of both of us bawling every time mealtime rolled around, my father showed up at the hospital bearing Guinness. He'd discussed the problem with a nurse he knew—which for a man of his generation showed just how worried he was—and she'd suggested I try drinking some Guinness, a traditional remedy for nursing mothers. I'd never imagined that my first alcoholic indulgence in months would be a lukewarm can of Guinness choked down under my dad's watchful eye (and out of the watchful eye of the nurses). A sort of calm settled over me, and I felt more relaxed about the whole situation. While I'm not endorsing alcohol as a nursing aid, anxiousness around breastfeeding can make the whole process more fraught and can affect milk supply.

Basically, drinking alcohol while breastfeeding is all a matter of timing. As a rule, postponing breastfeeding for two hours after having one drink will minimize your baby's exposure to alcohol—two hours is the minimum amount of time it takes to eliminate alcohol from the body. If you have one drink, the equivalent of one beer, one small glass of wine, or one ounce of hard alcohol, right after you finish breastfeeding, it should be mostly out of your system by your next breastfeeding session, unless you have a super-frequent feeder.

If you want to plan a bit of a bust-out, you can "pump and dump" your milk so you don't affect your milk supply as you would if you skipped a feeding entirely, and your baby can have some pre-pumped breast milk or an alternative. Of course, a little may go a long way after nine months of abstinence, so busting out may truly mean just a drink or two.

CAFFEINE

When you're breastfeeding and you haven't slept for more than two hours in a row for what seems like forever, is it cruel and unusual punishment to deny yourself any caffeine, or is it best for baby? The reality is too much caffeine in your breast milk may cause irritability and poor sleep in your baby, and who wants that? Health Canada's current guidelines suggest breastfeeding women not exceed 300 mg of caffeine a day. The good news is, that's approximately two to three cups of coffee, depending on how it's brewed, and six cups of tea, which should be enough to keep the edge off. You can also enjoy moderate amounts of chocolate without fear of harming your baby.

39

CIGARETTES

Though you may have been able to give up smoking while you were pregnant, you may be impatient to start up again now that your baby is born. But this isn't a good idea for a number of reasons (not the least of which is your health).

First, when you smoke, the nicotine and chemicals in the cigarette end up in your milk. Smoking 10 or more cigarettes a day could lead to irritability, diarrhea, vomiting, and poor weight gain in your baby. As well, you may have problems with your milk production. And finally, smoking around your baby will increase her risk for sudden infant death syndrome, not to mention asthma and other respiratory disorders, and lung cancer.

If you can't do without an occasional cigarette, have it right after you finish breastfeeding to try to limit the amount of nicotine and chemicals you pass on to your baby. Don't smoke around her, and anyone in your life who smokes should not do it around you and your baby.

THAT'S TOXIC

As we become more aware of the environmental damage from toxic substances, we're also becoming more aware of the damage within us from those same toxins. Toxins can kill or damage nerve and brain cells, and some are endocrine disrupters that interfere with normal hormonal activity.

Chemical residues accumulate in your body fat, which is in turn used to produce breast milk, so breast milk does transmit those chemicals and toxins to your baby. While you may panic and take this to mean your breast milk is toxic to your baby, that's not the case. Because breast milk contains substances that help children develop stronger immune systems and gives protection against environmental pollutants and pathogens, breast milk is still the best option for helping limit the damage caused by exposure to these substances.

The prevalent chemicals appearing in breast milk are called persistent organic pollutants (POPs). These are manufactured chemicals like DDT and other pesticides; PCBs (polychlorinated biphenyls); dioxins and PBDEs (polybrominated diphenyl ethers). Unlike toxins such as lead, POPs build up in our fatty tissue.

Formula is not a toxin-free alternative. Cow's-milk formulas can contain lead and aluminium from milk processing as well as bisphenol A (BPA) which is a lacquer used to coat metal containers such as food cans, and is an endocrine disrupter. They also contains phthalates, which are organic chemicals used as plasticizers that may also be endocrine disrupters.

While it takes many years to reduce the toxic burden in your body, here are some tips to help reduce toxic exposure during pregnancy and while breastfeeding:

- Avoid gasoline and dry-cleaning fumes. If you dry-clean your clothes, remove the plastic bags as soon as possible and air your clothes outside.
- Avoid fumes from paint, nail-polish removers, glue, and furniture strippers. Avoid installing new carpet or synthetic wood furniture as they also emit potentially hazardous gases. If it's impossible to avoid these completely, make sure you keep your home well ventilated.
- Remove lead paint from your home before you get pregnant. If you are already pregnant, breastfeeding,

or have a very young child, hire a certified lead contractor to remove the existing paint and repaint. Vacate your home completely until the process is complete.
- Avoid pesticide treatments, such as those for woodworm or rot.
- Don't eat fish that are high in mercury, such as shark, swordfish, and tilefish (see pages 31 to 32).
- In general, choose your foods from lower down the food chain, meaning more vegetables and grains and less meat.

ALL ORGANIC ALL THE TIME?

Unborn babies, infants, and children are those most vulnerable to pesticides and chemicals in their diets—and thus in breast milk. Does this mean a pregnant or breastfeeding mother must eat only organic food? Aside from the sometimes prohibitive cost of organic food, and the fact that it's not always widely available, not all organic food is created equal. In the following pages, I've identified which foods are best organic and those that aren't necessarily worth the money, and why.

Grain Products

Wheat and oatmeal are more likely to be contaminated with pesticide residue than barley or rice, so if you can, buy organic wheat- and oat-based products such as flour, pasta, and bread. If you can find organic rice for a good price it's also a worthwhile investment. Organic cereals for grown-ups are also good choices; however children's organic cereals are usually not fortified with vitamins and minerals like conventional cereals, so read the packaging carefully.

42

Vegetables and Fruit

The Environmental Working Group, an environmental watch-dog group in the United States, has identified the following vegetables and fruit as the top 12 most likely to be contaminated with pesticide and herbicide residue (in alphabetical order): apples, bell peppers, celery, cherries, grapes (imported), lettuce, nectarines, peaches, pears, potatoes, spinach, and strawberries. Conversely, the following are the 12 least likely to be contaminated: asparagus, avocados, bananas, broccoli, cabbage, corn, kiwi fruit, mangos, onions, papayas, pineapples, and peas. If organic vegetables and fruit don't fit your budget or are hard to find, regular vegetables and fruit are still an important part of any diet. Washing your produce well and peeling it can cut down on the amount of contaminants you eat, although peeling also cuts down on the fibre and nutrients.

Dairy

Unlike milk in the United States, Canadian milk does not contain the suspected carcinogen synthetic bovine somatotropin (BST), so it is "safer" than regular milk in the States. However, a UK study showed that organic milk contained more omega-3 fatty acids than non-organic milk, and significantly more vitamin E and beta carotene, probably a result of feeding differences between organic and conventional production. If you can afford it, organic milk is an excellent choice for breastfeeding mothers, their babies, and for your children when they start drinking cow's milk.

43

Protein

It costs farmers a lot more to raise organic meat and poultry, and that cost is passed on to the consumer; however here's an area where if you can buy organic it's worth it. Aside from being raised on chemical-free feed—and given no growth hormones, antibiotics, or animal-based feeds—organic meats are higher in omega-3s and lower in fat, while organic eggs are higher in omega-3s and beta carotene. If you cannot afford organic meat and poultry, natural meats that are raised without hormones or antibiotics are the next best choice.

FENDING OFF FUSSINESS

Mums are often told that their babies will react to their milk if they eat garlic or spicy foods, but all the experts agree that no foods should be banned from a breastfeeding mum's diet. Although it's normal for your baby to have fussy periods during the first three months, some babies develop colic or gas when their mums eat certain foods. And a mother faced with a colicky or fussy baby is willing to try anything to soothe her little one. Although you might think that gas-creating foods like beans, onions, and broccoli are likely culprits, current research shows that the main foods that affect your baby are dairy, eggs, wheat, and nuts—coincidentally the same most common foods to which babies develop allergies. If you notice that your baby gets fussy within two to four hours of your eating a certain food, try cutting it out of your diet for at least a week to clear your system and your baby's. Then reintroduce the food to see if it has the same effect. Don't try eliminating wheat, dairy, eggs, and nuts all in one go; it's too difficult to organize a healthy, well-balanced diet with all these restrictions.

44

Before cutting out an important food group be sure to consult your health care provider or a registered dietitian.

ALLERGIES

If food allergies run in your family, the best way to prevent your baby from developing them is to exclusively breastfeed her for at least the first six months. Breastfed babies just aren't exposed to as many allergens as formula-fed babies and that lessens their risk of developing allergies. Colostrum, the initial milk produced when breastfeeding begins, is especially rich in antibodies and coats baby's intestines to protect against potential allergens. By six months, a baby's immune system is functional, if immature, and capable of producing the antibodies necessary to defend against allergens.

If severe food allergies run in your family, you might also want to consider avoiding the foods that children are commonly

A Mum's Story

My daughter Odessa was born shortly before Christmas, the season of amazing foods and wonderful flavours.
I put together a gorgeous cheese board for visitors to the house and sat tucking into some fabulous blue cheese that I just couldn't stop eating. The flavour must have migrated into my breast milk because poor Odessa could barely stand the taste. The poor little girl was so hungry that she ate, but I can still remember her heartbroken cries as she took each gulp.

—*Emma, mother of two*

45

allergic to, such as nuts, milk, and eggs, while breastfeeding. Studies have shown that this could help prevent or delay your child from developing allergies.

If you suspect allergies in your baby because they run in your family, or because your baby seems to have a lot of skin irritation, diarrhea, vomiting, or restless sleep, it's important to be careful when introducing solid foods. Your health care professional or a registered dietitian will be able to give you some guidance, and there are many websites and books with specific information on allergies and children (see Appendix D, page 173).

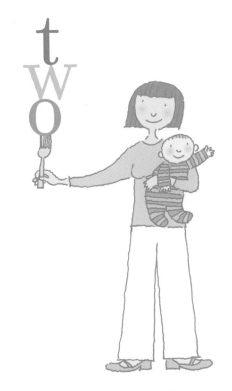

two

HEALTHY EATING SURVIVAL GUIDE

4

STOCKING UP: GETTING YOUR
KITCHEN BABY-READY

During my first pregnancy, I was relatively realistic about what the early weeks of parenthood would be like. I knew that the hours spent counting my baby's perfect little toes and exclaiming over her tiny fingernails would be offset by the many more hours spent pacing the floor trying to calm her cries. But it wasn't until she was born that I truly understood what the term "sleep deprivation" meant (and why it's been used as a form of torture by dictatorial regimes). I was constantly hungry but too exhausted to do more than open a tin of sardines and fork them into my mouth while standing at the kitchen counter. If anyone had suggested I plan a week's worth of meals, make a comprehensive grocery list, go shopping, and spend the afternoon cooking, hysterical tears would have ensued.

At the weekend-long, intensive prenatal class that my husband and I attended, the midwife who taught us advised

49

us to stock up our freezer with meals before my due date, but I was too overcome by films of childbirth and talk of episiotomies to pay her much heed. And besides, the last trimester of my pregnancy took place during the sweltering months of summer when standing in a hot kitchen didn't do much for my swollen ankles. I did manage to freeze a few entrees, but after Madeleine was born, my husband and I had no option but to depend on the kindness of family, friends, and takeout, which isn't the healthiest or most economical alternative. While you can take much of the advice you're given before your baby's born with a grain of salt, stop and listen to anyone who suggests you channel your nesting instincts into stocking up your freezer, pantry, and refrigerator before your bundle of joy arrives.

Like all the baby books that include handy lists of all the "equipment" you'll need to take good care of your baby, in this chapter I'll give you lists of what to stock up on in the kitchen to take good care of yourself. Trust me, having an ample supply of food on hand will be a lifesaver while you're stumbling through the first weeks of parenthood, hungry yet housebound by leaky breasts or a colicky baby.

THE RIGHT STUFF

Now that your needs will be changing a bit, it's time to take stock of your kitchen equipment and assess whether there's anything you might want to buy. Having the right tools makes preparing, cooking, and storing food that much easier. If you haven't been in the habit of stocking large supplies of food, you might want to invest in a freezer. While the refrigerator freezer can accommodate quite a number of meals if

50

you pack skillfully, a deep freezer will hold a lot more and will allow you to be a little more lackadaisical about arranging the containers. You might also want to think about getting a free-standing cupboard if you don't have a lot of cupboard space in your kitchen. Alternatively, you could use a closet or shelf space in another area of your home, like the basement, to store extra cans of food and supplies. Buying in bulk and stocking up will not only mean fewer and shorter trips to the supermarket but also may save you some money. Here is a list of the basic equipment you will need to make and freeze the recipes in this book as well as the majority of your favourite recipes.

3- to 4-inch paring knife
10-inch chef's knife
10-inch carving knife
8-inch serrated knife
2 cutting boards: 1 for vegetables and fruit; 1 for meat, poultry, and fish
Set of 3 graduated mixing bowls
10-inch non-stick frying pan
10-inch ovenproof sauté pan with a heavy bottom
1-quart saucepan with fitted lid
2 ½-quart saucepan with fitted lid
8–12 quart stockpot with fitted lid
Large casserole dish with lid
Small casserole dish with lid
1–2 12-cup muffin pans
1 9- x 13-inch cake pan
1–2 9- x 5-inch loaf pans

1–2 baking sheets
Blender and/or food processor
Bottle opener
Can opener
Citrus juicer
Colander
Corkscrew
Electric mixer
Funnel
Garlic press
Grater
Meat thermometer
Nutcracker
Potato masher
Rolling pin
Rubber scraper
Set of measuring spoons
Set of measuring cups for dry ingredients

2-cup glass measuring cup for
  liquid ingredients
Sifter
Slotted spoon
Soup ladle
Spatulas, 1–2
Strainer, large
Strainer, small
Tongs
Vegetable peeler

Whisk
Wooden spoons
Zester
Tight-lidded plastic
  refrigerator/freezer storage
  containers in all sizes
Plastic freezer bags
Aluminum foil
Heavy-duty plastic wrap

THE FREEZER

Frozen food won't keep forever, so don't start stocking your postnatal freezer until a month or two before your due date. Here's a handy reference chart for how long cooked food will last in your freezer:

Food Type	Freezer Life
Cooked meat, stews, egg, or vegetable dishes	2–3 months
Cooked poultry and fish	4–6 months
Soups	4 months
Gravy and meat stock	2–3 months

There are two ways to go about filling your freezer with postnatal meals. One is to devote a weekend here and there to cooking. The other, which may seem less overwhelming—and easier on your back and swollen feet—is to double up on the meals you prepare during the weeks leading up to your due date and put the extras in the freezer. Although it will take

52

slightly longer to chop more vegetables and to bring larger quantities of soups and stews to a simmer, it will still be much quicker than making the same recipe on two or three different nights. This big-batch method requires recognizing which recipes will double easily and freeze well. Here's a list of the freezer-friendly entree recipes in this book:

Asparagus or Broccoli Frittata (page 130)
Ham, Cheese, and Mushroom Frittata (page 132)
Pollo Salsa Verde (page 142)
White Chili (page 144)
AJ's Whole Wheat Mac 'n' Cheese (page 146)
Salmon and Spinach Quiche (page 154)
Andrew's Spaghetti Sauce (page 156)
Garlic Ginger Sweet Potato Soup (page 158)
Lentil Soup (page 160)
Beef Stew (page 162)

If you choose to power cook over a weekend, here's a plan of action:

POWER COOK WEEKEND
Day One
• Choose the recipes you'd like to make. Aside from being freezable, they should also vary in type and taste so you don't end up with a freezer full of variations on spaghetti sauce. Choose three or four different dishes and ensure they don't all require the same cooking method; you could run out of oven space or burners.

53

- Make sure you have all the necessary equipment to prepare the recipes as well as the storage containers for freezing.
- Make your shopping list, organizing it into categories the way your supermarket is laid out; for example, fresh produce, deli counter, breads, canned goods, dairy case, frozen foods, and so on.
- Go grocery shopping.
- Start prepping: wash the vegetables and cut them and the meat and/or poultry up for cooking the next day.

Day Two
- Put on your favourite music and get out all the ingredients you'll need. Be sure to empty the dishwasher so you can load it as you go.
- Start cooking the recipe that takes the longest amount of time, then the recipe that takes the second longest, up until the recipe that takes the least.
- Save time by combining the same steps in different recipes. If you're sautéing onion for one dish, sauté enough for all the dishes you're making that day. Likewise, brown all the ground beef you'll be using.
- Remember that your dish will get extra cooking when it's reheated, so take it off the burner or out of the oven a few minutes before it's completely done.
- Wash as you go to make cleanup more manageable and so you don't end up with a huge, teetering pile of dirty dishes. (Or better yet, get a spouse or sous-chef to do them.)

DISHING IT OUT

It's important to cool food as quickly as possible to prevent bacterial growth. Don't put hot food in your refrigerator or freezer; instead, divide the food into smaller quantities in shallow containers and cool to just about room temperature, within two hours. Then freeze it immediately, for safety reasons and because food frozen at its freshest tastes better. Food expands when it's frozen, so fill containers to only within a half-inch from the top. Seal it with a tightly fitting lid, and use a permanent marker to identify the contents, reheating instructions, and the date. Or better yet, use the charts on pages 52 and 57 to calculate its best-before date and record that on the label so you won't have to do the calculations when you're rushing to grab something to thaw for dinner. Pop the containers in the freezer in a single layer so they freeze as quickly as possible. Once they are frozen, you can stack them to optimize space. Your freezer should be set at -18°C.

Running Out of Dishes?

You might be tempted to stick your baked lasagna in its casserole dish in the freezer, but what if you need the dish for another freezable meal? Try this trick: Line the dish with aluminum foil before filling. Freeze the finished casserole, then simply lift the food out of the dish and pop it in a freezer bag. When you're ready to reheat, remove the food from the freezer, peel away the aluminum foil, and put the frozen block of food back in the casserole dish to defrost in the refrigerator.

55

If you're really organized, keep a list on your computer or taped to the side of your freezer listing its inventory. Keeping it updated will prevent you from ending up with nothing but five dishes of macaroni and cheese or discovering a stash of past-its-prime food buried beneath a layer of permafrost.

FREEZER FUNDAMENTALS

In addition to all your homemade meals, it's a good idea to keep a supply of multipurpose basics in your freezer so you won't be caught out. With the following list of frozen foods on hand you'll always be able to whip up a quick lunch or dinner.

Bread (including whole-grain loaves, pita, tortillas, bagels, and English muffins)
Chicken (boneless, skinless breasts are the most versatile)
Fish fillets
Fruit (including berries and sliced peaches for adding to oatmeal, smoothies, and muffins)
Fruit juice concentrates
Ground beef, turkey, or chicken
Ice cream
Milk
Nitrate-free bacon

Pie shells
Pizza crusts
Sausages
Shrimp (precooked)
Shrimp (uncooked, shelled and deveined)
Steaks and chops
Vegetables (including spinach, edamame, corn, peas and mixed vegetables)
Veggie, beef, or chicken burgers
Wheat bran
Wheat germ

While frozen foods can be stored indefinitely, they taste better—and are safer—if you eat them within the following timelines.

Food Type	Freezer Life
Bacon	1 month
Bagels	2 months
Beef roasts and steak	4 months
Bread	3 months
Chicken and turkey, pieces	6 months
Chicken and turkey, whole	1 year
Fatty fish (salmon, tuna, etc.)	2 months
Fruit	4–6 months
Fruit juice concentrate	6–12 months
Ground meat	2–3 months
Lamb roasts and chops	8–12 months
Lean deli ham or turkey	1–2 months
Lean fish (cod, flounder, etc.)	6 months
Milk	3 months
Pork roasts and chops	8–12 months
Sausage	1–2 months
Scallops, Shrimp	2–4 months
Shellfish (clams, crab, lobster)	2–4 months
Tortillas, pita	4 months
Veal roasts and chops	2–4 months
Vegetables	8–12 months
Yogurt	1–2 months

THE PANTRY

The last couple of weeks before your due date is a good time to start thinking about stocking your postnatal pantry. You know you're going to need items like pasta and chicken broth, so why not buy multiple quantities now when you have the time for shopping and putting away groceries? While you're at it, buy supplies of household basics such as toilet paper, paper towel, laundry detergent, and dish liquid. The following list includes all the shelf-stable foods you'll need to make all the recipes in this book. If you have any quick and easy recipe standbys you plan to make use of when baby arrives, add the ingredients you'll need to this list as well as any items you use on a regular basis.

Pantry Staples

Cooking Oils
Canola oil
Flaxseed oil
Olive oil
Sesame oil

Canned Food
Anchovies
Artichoke hearts
Black beans
Chicken broth (low sodium)
Chickpeas (garbanzo beans)
Kidney beans (red and white)
Navy beans
Olives
Romano beans
Sardines
Tomatoes (diced or crushed)
Tuna, light

Sauces and Condiments
Balsamic vinegar

Curry paste
Dijon mustard
Low-sodium stock (beef, chicken, or vegetable)
Marinara pasta sauce
Peanut, cashew, or almond butter
Pesto
Plain tomato sauce
Red wine vinegar
Salsa
Salsa verde (green salsa)
Soy sauce
Sweet chili sauce
Tahini
White vinegar
Worcestershire sauce

Grains and Pasta
Barley
Brown rice
Dried lentils
Orecchiette, penne, or fusilli pasta

58

Pasta shells, small
Spaghetti
Whole wheat elbow macaroni

Baking Sundries
All Bran™ cereal
Baking powder
Baking soda
Brown sugar
Cornmeal
Cornstarch
Corn syrup
Flour
Granulated white sugar
Honey
Maple syrup
Molasses
Quick-cooking oats
Steel-cut oats or large-flake
    rolled oats

Spices
Basil (dried)
Bay leaves
Black peppercorns
Cayenne
Chili powder
Cinnamon
Cumin
Ginger (ground)
Nutmeg
Oregano (dried)
Paprika
Sage (dried)
Salt
Small dried red chilies
Thyme (dried)

Cooking Spirits
Dry sherry
Red wine

MAKE SNACKS A STAPLE

When your baby arrives, you'll be so caught up in feeding him that you may feel you have no time to feed yourself. In addition to eating regular meals, snacking throughout the day is a good way to keep your energy levels up—and some days, snacks will be the only way you'll manage to get enough to eat.

Stock up on foods that will make healthy, nutrient-rich snacks with little to no preparation and that can be eaten one-handed. Many of the most popular prepared snack foods are full of sugar and/or trans fats, and the energy boost you get from these empty calories will be brief, leaving you craving more.

59

If someone's offered to throw you a shower and asks your opinion on themes, why not suggest food? Okay, it's not as cute as baby booties, but there's no reason attendees can't throw a few of those into the mix as well. The hostess can ask each guest to bring you a freezable entree labelled with cooking instructions—a copy of the recipe is a nice addition too.

Nutrition labelling shows what you're getting per serving in terms of calories and nutrients. "Per serving" is key, as you may be surprised to find that a serving of potato chips has only 120 calories but the chip manufacturer counts 10 potato chips as a serving. Have you ever managed to eat only 10? Or maybe the package advertises "low in fat" but doesn't go on to say "but with *tons* of sugar!"

Try to steer clear of foods that contain artificial preservatives, colours, and flavours, and hydrogenated and trans fats. It is now becoming mandatory for manufacturers in Canada to list trans fat contents on packaging. Government and industry are also collaborating to reduce the levels of trans fats in foods. Fortunately, manufacturers have realized that shoppers are becoming much more savvy and particular about what they buy, and there are now "trans fat free" versions of many prepared foods. Seek them out; they're better for you and your baby.

And don't just look at the label, *look* at what you're buying. As a rule, the more your food is in its natural, unprocessed state, the better it is for you. Day-glo orange cheezies are highly processed and practically nutrient-free—the diet equivalent of entertainment television. But you know that. The trickiest foods to get the real scoop on are those that seem healthy when they aren't. If you check the nutrition label on your multigrain bread, you may find that it's made of 95 percent refined flour with a bit of whole wheat thrown in. And that "made with real juice" drink you buy does contain real juice, but only about 10 percent. And then there are the many guises of sugar, such

A Mum's Story

After my first baby was born, I was soon on a first-name, pretty much topless basis with our postman who rang our doorbell almost daily with a special delivery, usually while I was in the midst of breastfeeding. We had a constant stream of visitors bringing by lovely little gifts for her, beautiful onesies, plush toys, and soft blankets—our nursery was overflowing. And then one day a friend who had her first baby right after we did came to visit and brought with her a huge cellophane-wrapped basket from a local upscale market. It was filled with treats for me. "I tried to buy things you could eat with one hand," she explained. The basket contained little thumbprint cookies baked with an ancient, fibrous grain; premade smoothies; hummus with baby carrots; trail mix; and cheeses with gourmet crackers. It was such a nice treat to have someone thinking of just me and was one of the best gifts I received.

—Annemarie, mother of two

Dark chocolate that contains at least 70 percent cocoa solids is good for you (in small amounts, anyway). It's not only a source of polyphenols, the same type of antioxidant found in red wine, but it also contains flavonoids, which are beneficial for your heart.

as dextrose, sucrose, and corn syrup. Paying attention to nutrition labels and understanding what they mean is an important step in eating well. But you don't have to be a saint—a few judiciously chosen treats among all the healthy stuff will satisfy your cravings. A small square of good-quality dark chocolate or a single scoop of ice cream might be just the flavour hit you need to get you through a rough patch. After all, research has shown that if you crave something but eat everything else in an attempt to avoid it, you may end up eating more calories than you would have in the first place, without killing the craving. So go ahead and add some dark chocolate or your favourite ice cream to the following list of healthy snack supplies.

Shelf-Stable Snack Staples

Baked, trans-fat-free tortilla chips
Bottled salsa
Canned chickpeas
Canned fruit in juice or water
Canned legumes, such as kidney
  beans and black beans
Canned light tuna
Canned sardines
Dried fruit, such as apricots, cranberries, dates, figs, and raisins

Dry-roasted soy nuts
Nut butters, such as peanut, cashew,
  and almond
Trans-fat-free whole-grain crackers,
  such as whole wheat or rye crisps
Unsweetened applesauce
Whole-grain cereal with little or
  no sugar

Perishable Snack Staples

Because these items will not keep for long, buy only what you will eat in a week.

Apples	Low-fat sandwich meats, such
Avocados	as turkey, lean ham, and roast
Bananas	beef
Bell peppers	Nuts, such as almonds, hazelnuts,
Cantaloupe	and walnuts
Carrots	Oranges
Celery	Papaya
Cheese	Pumpkin seeds
Cherry or grape tomatoes	Soy milk
Cottage cheese	Sunflower seeds
Cream cheese	Whole-grain bread
Cucumbers	Whole-grain English muffins
Eggs	Whole-grain pita
Frozen edamame	Whole-grain tortillas
Low-fat dips	Yogurt
Low-fat milk	

Here are a few healthy snacking ideas:

- Whole-grain cereal with low-fat milk or soy milk
- Whole-grain crackers with low-fat cheese or peanut butter
- Tortilla chips with salsa
- Low-fat nachos: Spread tortilla chips out on a baking dish, sprinkle with rinsed and drained canned red kidney or black beans and cheese, and bake in oven or microwave until cheese is melted. Add salsa or guacamole on the side.
- Quesadilla: Place a whole wheat tortilla in a non-stick skillet over medium heat. Sprinkle with cheese. Fold tortilla over, and heat until tortilla is golden and cheese is melted. Top with salsa or guacamole.

63

- Tina's Hummus (see recipe on page 110) with baby carrots, cucumbers, and whole wheat pita
- Guacamole (see recipe on page 109) with bell pepper strips, grape tomatoes, and tortilla chips
- Handful of dried fruit, nuts, or seeds
- Unsweetened applesauce, yogurt, and cinnamon
- A piece of fresh fruit
- Celery sticks filled with nut butter, or cream or cottage cheese
- Apple slices with peanut butter
- Canned light tuna or sardines on crackers or toast
- Slice of lean deli ham and slice of Swiss cheese, rolled up
- Slice of lean roast beef and lettuce leaf, rolled up
- Handful of soy nuts
- Boiled edamame with a light sprinkling of salt
- A hard-boiled egg
- Low-fat cottage cheese with some canned fruit
- A glass of low-fat milk
- A sandwich
- Homemade trail mix: Combine 1 cup raisins, 1 cup nuts, 1 cup dried apricots or cranberries, and $\frac{1}{2}$ cup sunflower seeds in a large resealable plastic bag.
- Fruit with Honey Yogurt Dip: Blend together 1 cup of plain or vanilla low-fat yogurt, $\frac{1}{4}$ cup honey, and $\frac{1}{2}$ tsp cinnamon.

The following recipes can also be prepared ahead of time and frozen for delicious, healthy snacks:

Oatmeal Pancakes (page 90)
Eva's Energy Bars (page 92)
Lemon Blueberry Muffins (page 94)
Carrot Raisin Muffins (page 96)
Fruit Muffins (page 98)
Three-Grain Blueberry Muffins (page 100)
Carrot Breakfast Bars (page 102)
Diane's Banana Bread (page 104)

GO GOURMET

It's unlikely you'll be doing a lot of fine dining in the early days of your baby's life, but why not add the occasional gourmet touch to your snacks? Treating yourself to some of the foods you missed out on while you were pregnant, like blue cheese and smoked salmon, will make you feel pampered—even if you're gulping down your snack on the go.

Marinated olives
Tapenade with gourmet crackers
Sun-dried tomatoes stuffed with anchovies
Cheeses such as brie and blue
Whole-wheat pretzels with spicy hot mustard
Smoked salmon, cream cheese, and capers on black bread
Prosciutto and cantaloupe
Cooked shrimp with cocktail sauce

Your pantry is full and your freezer is satisfyingly stocked with clearly labelled entrees and muffins. All this preparation will help you eat well and give you more time to sleep, shower, and spend time with your baby in the weeks ahead.

5

HOW TO COOK AND EAT WHEN YOU DON'T HAVE TIME TO COOK OR EAT

Nothing you do before the arrival of your baby can truly prepare you for all the peaks and valleys of life as a new parent. No matter how much sleep you banked during your last trimester, you're bound to be exhausted by Junior's marathon schedule, and no matter what you might have tried to toughen up your nipples, you may need some adjusting to your wee baby's powerful suction—which probably rivals that of the latest and greatest vacuum model! And really, there was nothing that could have prepared you for the roller coaster of emotions you'll be riding as a new mum. One moment you'll be feeling overwhelmed with love for your child and the next you'll be sobbing over the loss of your pre-baby waistline and your pre-baby life. Mothers' groups are a great excuse to get out of the house and talk about your fears, worries, and wonder with other mums. Sharing your experiences will also help you to recognize that all your emotions are perfectly natural and felt by most other mothers too.

Realizing you're not the only mum who ever leaked milk in the grocery store or gave up on reusable diapers and switched to disposables for convenience, will help you go easy on yourself.

If you enjoyed an orderly life and home before baby, it's time to readjust your expectations and priorities. You simply won't be able to maintain your usual cleaning, cooking, and self-care routines. You'll need to re-evaluate and be realistic about what's possible to accomplish in a day and pare down your jobs and responsibilities. It's hard, but here's how one mother I know summed it up: "I just had to really lower all my standards and then everything was fine and I wasn't so stressed out by all the mess and dirt." Here are some suggestions for how you might lower your standards and make your life simpler:

- Organize the house for convenience and function, not for appearance. For example, set up an area or two where you will be breastfeeding and keep a pillow, blanket, burp cloths, bottles of water, snacks, and anything else that you'll need there.
- Use paper plates and cups to minimize cleanup.
- Try to put things away as you use them to keep down clutter.
- Keep ongoing lists of items you need and errands and jobs that need doing. These lists are also something you can hand to your husband when he gets home or to another family member or friend who offers help.
- Don't be afraid to accept help or to ask for it. This is not the time to put on a brave face and pretend you've got everything under control—unless you do, in which case tell us how you do it! Family and friends are usually

more than willing to help where they can, either by running an errand or watching the baby for an hour while you go out.

- Instead of doing the laundry yourself, send it out to the cleaners.
- Hire someone to give the house a weekly cleaning or to do any of the chores you can't get around to.

Some of the suggestions above might seem extravagant to you, but they are only for the short term as you settle into your new routine, and could make a huge difference to your quality of life and peace of mind. After all, your priorities right now are to look after your baby, get as much rest as possible, and eat a healthy diet.

A Mum's Story

One day when I was very pregnant, I was crossing the street when an old man yelled at me, "Paper plates!" I thought he was just insane—that is until the baby arrived. By day five we had 100 paper plates in the cupboard and a big black garbage bag in the corner. When my friend Anne was pregnant with her second child, she decided to pay attention to the old man too. She had 500 paper plates and cups waiting for her in the kitchen when she came home with her new baby. It was the best advice we'd ever heard.

—Sheila, mother of two

RELY ON THE MEALS YOU'VE FROZEN

When you pull a meal out of the freezer, defrost it in the fridge if you've got enough time. Otherwise, defrost it under cold running water or in the microwave. Food defrosted in the microwave should be eaten immediately. Food that has been frozen should be eaten within three days of being removed from the freezer.

Reheat solid food to at least 165°F and do it fast. Reheat soups and sauces to a rolling boil. Don't reheat your already reheated leftovers, much as it may pain you to discard them. No matter how great your sense of smell has become during and after pregnancy, neither your nose, eyes, nor tastebuds are an accurate judge of the safety of your food. If in doubt, throw it out.

THINK OUTSIDE THE (LUNCH) BOX

Don't think that your meals have to fit conventional standards of what constitutes a breakfast or dinner. Who says that leftover soup or rice pudding can't be enjoyed at breakfast or that a sandwich or scrambled eggs aren't a perfectly respectable dinner? You need to keep yourself well fuelled, and that may mean being flexible about what you eat, and eating several small meals and healthy snacks throughout the day when you can't manage to sit down for a proper meal.

After Madeleine was born, I discovered that woman can survive on muffins alone—well almost. My favourites were Lemon Blueberry Muffins (see recipe on page 94) because they were quick to make and eat, and very tasty. I'd make a double batch, leave a few out, and freeze the rest. On my way out of the house, I'd grab one from the freezer, pop it into my diaper bag, and it was ready to eat when I arrived at my destination.

Easy Reading for Mum

Here are a few suggestions for a little light
reading about motherhood that will reassure you
that you aren't the only one who's yet to perfect
the art of the play date.

Fiction:

Mommy-Track Mysteries by Ayelet Waldman

Baby Proof by Emily Giffin

I Don't Know How She Does It by Allison Pearson

The Wives of Bath by Wendy Holden

24-Karat Kids by Judy Goldstein &
Sebastian Stuart

Non-Fiction:

*The Three-Martini Playdate: A Practical Guide to Happy
Parenting* by Christie Mellor

Operating Instructions: A Journal of My Son's First Year
by Anne Lamott

*Momfidence!: An Oreo Never Killed Anybody
and Other Secrets of Happier Parenting* by
Paula Spencer

Snacking can be done one-handed while nursing or
pushing a stroller. Sometimes getting you and baby out of the
house to see friends may seem more important for your men-
tal health than actually eating, but munching a toasted English muffin with peanut butter on your way to your play date

A Mum's Story

Sabine was ten days old and had decided that given the choice between sleeping or feeding, she'd take feeding. She fed non-stop for hours on end. She'd stop only to throw up and then start again like some crazed Roman binger. Consequently I was a prisoner of the couch and starving. My husband had to feed me in between bites of his food and I got very upset if he took two bites and I only got one. I'm really not sure what I ate that month other than lots of cold hash browns and egg rolls.

—Frances, mother of two

ensures that you get to do both. See pages 63 to 65 for plenty of healthy snack ideas.

SIMPLIFIED MEAL PLANNING, SHOPPING, AND COOKING

It's a sad certainty that you will eventually empty your freezer, and that's why the recipes in this book were developed with new mums in mind. Out of necessity, I tested them very thoroughly after Lucy, my second daughter, was born. They are all easy to prepare; some can be made in 10 minutes or less, while others can be assembled in minutes and then left to simmer on the stove while you attend to your baby. On pages 56 to 59, I listed all the ingredients that could be stored in your pantry and freezer to make the recipes in this book. On the next page is a list of the perishable ingredients you will need. Some of these are also listed in the perishable snack staples on page 63.

72

Produce Aisle

Asparagus
Avocados
Baby spinach
Bananas
Bell peppers
Broccoli
Carrots
Celery
Eggplant
Fresh basil
Fresh cilantro
Fresh parsley
Fresh thyme
Garlic
Gingeroot
Green onions
Leeks
Lemons (for juice and zest)
Lettuce
Limes (for juice and zest)
Mushrooms
Onions
Oranges (for juice and zest)
Peas (fresh and frozen)
Potatoes
Red onions
Soft tofu
Sweet potatoes
Tomatoes
Zucchini

Bakery

Crusty whole-grain bread

Whole wheat pita bread
Whole wheat tortillas

Dairy

Brie
Cheddar
Cottage cheese (dry)
Eggs
Feta
Goat cheese
Gouda
Half-and-half cream
Milk
Monterey Jack
Plain yogurt
Parmesan (fresh grated)
Ricotta
Soy milk
Vanilla yogurt

Poultry, Meat, and Seafood

(Some of these items may already
  be in your freezer.)
Beef steaks
Chicken
Chicken breasts (skinless, boneless)
Ground beef (lean)
Lean cooked ham
Pancetta
Salami
Salmon steaks
Shrimp (uncooked, shelled, and
  deveined)
Stewing beef (lean)

73

Start getting organized by planning the upcoming week's meals based on what's happening and when you'll have help in the kitchen or more time to cook. Use a meal from the freezer on a night you know you won't have much cooking time, and make a double batch of stew or spaghetti sauce on the weekend when your husband is home to help out. Depending on your husband's culinary skills and schedule, you could take turns cooking each evening—or leave the cooking entirely up to him (but then why would you be reading this chapter?).

Once you have a list of meals you plan to make, complete your grocery list. Cut corners by buying pre-chopped vegetables, prewashed salad mixes, and grated cheese. Also, buy shelf-stable staples in bulk; why buy one can of tomatoes when you can buy five? Have your butcher cut all your meat and poultry so it's ready for the pan. Find out if there is an online grocery delivery service in your neighbourhood and use it. These services usually allow you to create a staples list, which will save you even more time each week and help twig your baby-fuddled brain to things you need. Alternatively, you might want to do a weekly shop on a weeknight or weekend when you can fly solo. After the first six weeks or so with

> ## Get Out and About
>
> An hour or two away from your crazy life can work wonders, so have your husband, relative, or sitter watch your baby and either plan a regular activity that you enjoy such as a yoga class or a book club, or just go for a walk in the park, window shop with a latte in hand, or go see a movie that isn't rated G.

Madeleine, I liked to go for a daily stroll with her to the local
shops to buy fresh food.

COOKING

You have your recipes planned out and your groceries bought,
and now you need to find the time to cook. I was lucky
enough to have a baby who, quite early on, settled into a routine of a morning nap, an early afternoon nap, and a late afternoon nap, and I took advantage of it. I used her nap times
for showering, sending emails, tidying up, and cooking. Once
she went down for her morning nap, I would whip up a batch
of muffins in about 10 to 15 minutes and pop them in the
oven. I'd jump in the shower, and by the time I was done,
so were the muffins, which I'd enjoy with a cup of tea before

75

I was back on baby duty. Depending on how the afternoon would go, I'd prep and even cook dinner—particularly if it was something that could be left to simmer—during Madeleine's early afternoon nap. If I was doing a quick and easy dinner, I'd do the cooking or at least the prep during her third nap of the day.

Cooking with Two

Why not set up a play date for mums? If you each have a little one about the same age, schedule a morning or afternoon for cooking together. Each of you can plan and shop for one freezer-friendly, big-batch meal and then gather at one house to cook up a storm. Make sure you have, or bring, all the pots, pans, and freezer bags necessary, and whip up a couple of meals between naps and nursing. You'll each be set with a few different meals for the freezer, and as it's unlikely both kids will be totally in sync schedule-wise, there'll always be a spare pair of hands to turn off the oven, stir the soup, change a diaper, or sing lullabies. And there's bound to be some time for you to put up your feet, sip some tea, and trade tales of sleep deprivation and stretch marks.

This routine works well if you have a baby who's regular, but it all goes out the window if your baby doesn't settle nicely into a routine. If you can't plan anything around your little one's naps because they just aren't reliable, there's no reason not to do some cooking while your baby's awake. I had a lifesaving mobile that played a 20-minute rotation of classical music—Mozart makes you smarter, after all! My baby loved it and most mornings I'd lay her down to watch it, make a batch of oatmeal in the microwave, sprinkle it with nuts and brown sugar, and gulp it down as I watched her watch the rotating giraffes.

When you're ready to cook dinner, move your baby's play mat near the kitchen so she can see what you're up to, crank some tunes—yours or hers—and keep up a running commentary: "Now Mummy's chopping up carrots. You're going to eat carrots soon and I think you're going to like them. Do you know that when Mummy was little she ate so many carrots that the palms of her hands and the soles of her feet turned orange?" Okay, you may feel a tiny bit moronic, but just think, you'll be cooking, interacting, and fostering your baby's developing language skills all in one go, you multi-tasker you. Slings and baby carriers can work too unless you're involved in tasks that involve sizzling oil and only until baby starts to grab for that razor-sharp paring knife you're using on the potatoes. It helps to do all the nursing, diaper-changing, and prep work before you begin cooking. That way you're not trying to slice mushrooms, stir pasta, and calm a frantic baby all at the same time. Instead you can just stir the pasta and calm the baby—trust me, it makes a difference.

DIALING FOR FOOD

Of course, there will be days when you don't have the time, energy, ingredients, or inclination to cook. If you opt for someone else to show up at your door bearing dinner once in a

77

while, then by all means indulge in your favourite dishes. However, if ordering in is becoming a habit, here are a few tips on making healthier choices.

Pizza

Thin-crust pizza loaded with veggies is quite a healthy meal. If you have the option of choosing a whole wheat crust, that'll make it even better. Try choosing lower-fat toppings like ham, chicken, mushrooms, peppers, tomatoes, and artichokes rather than higher-fat toppings like bacon, sausage, salami, pepperoni, and olives, or at least mix them up a little. And go easy on the cheese.

Sushi

Sushi is a takeout star, and post-pregnancy you can indulge in all your favourites again. Sushi made without mayonnaise is better for you, so choose a tuna roll rather than a spicy tuna roll, which contains mayonnaise. If the spicy one is what you're craving, however, you might as well go for it, since sushi is still such a good choice.

Fast Food

Fast foods tend to be high in fat, calories, and sodium, and low in fibre and nutrients. In light of dropping sales, fast-food chains are trying to add healthier choices to their menus. Grilled chicken sandwiches, veggie burgers, salads, and yogurt cups are pretty good choices. If you must have fries then really, really enjoy them.

78

A Mum's Story

The kindest thing that happened in the first five
months with my baby was my friend Marni showed up
at the door around noon with a meal she had prepared,
complete with silverware, napkins, and china. She set
me a place at my own table, took my lovely lump of a
boy in her arms, and made sure I ate her homemade
soup, chicken, and pasta without interruption until I
was full. I still get weepy with gratitude when I think
about it.

I'm now the person at the party or family gathering
who relieves the new mother of her charge as she strug-
gles to juggle the baby and her plate. People assume I do
this because I am especially fond of babies, and there's
a morsel of truth in that, but it's really because I deeply
believe mothers need to be fed, and deserve to eat their
food while it's hot.

My youngest son is now 16 and 6 foot 6, and the fridge
gets raided most nights at midnight and again at two in
the morning. He's still a nocturnal eater. But he has been
known on occasion to get up early and make his mother
his own brand of Egg McMuffin for breakfast.

—*Anne, mother of two*

Indian

With Indian food the key is to limit deep-fried foods and
dishes cooked with cream sauces. Focus on dishes cooked in
tomato sauces.

79

Thai

Alas, many Thai dishes are made with coconut milk, which is quite high in saturated fat, so try not to indulge in them too often. You don't necessarily have to deprive yourself of your favourite dish, just make sure that the dishes you order don't all contain coconut or are deep-fried. Mix things up with healthy choices. Thai food also tends to be heavy on peanuts, so keep that in mind if you're worried about allergies.

Chinese

Find an MSG-free restaurant and mainly opt for dishes that are stir-fried, not deep-fried, and those that have lots of veggies such as steamed veggie dumplings or mu shu pork.

Italian

Words to avoid at Italian eateries are "breaded," "fried," and "deep-fried"; better choices are "broiled," "baked," "grilled," or "poached." Pastas with veggies and tomato sauces beat out lasagnas and pastas with cream sauces every time. As for garlic bread, well, what do you think?

Mexican

How can beans be bad for you? Well, when they're refried and served with sour cream and guacamole they're certainly not great. Try opting for veggie burritos, and have beans on the side that aren't refried. If you're tempted by nachos remember that an order of all-dressed, full-meal-deal nachos usually contains more than your day's recommended daily fat intake.

When you're ordering in or eating out it's also important to be aware of portion size. Try to save leftovers for next day's lunch if you think you have too much on your plate. If you're trying to make healthier choices when eating out, opt for food that's been baked, barbecued, broiled, charbroiled, grilled, poached, roasted, steamed, or stir-fried over anything battered, creamed, breaded, or deep-fried.

three

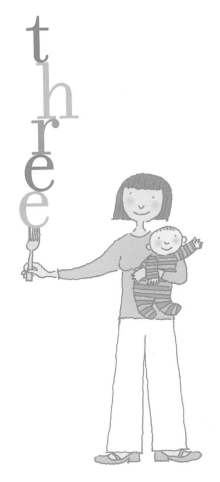

THE RECIPES

6

BREAKFASTS AND SNACKS

15 minutes or less

Basic Berry Smoothie

Start to finish time: 5 minutes

Prep time: 5 minutes

Smoothies are perfect for a quick breakfast or snack. When making this one for breakfast, double the recipe so you have another smoothie for a snack later. Just remember to give it a good stir before sipping.

1 ripe banana

$3/4$ cup frozen berries (blueberries, raspberries, strawberries, or a mix)

$1/2$ cup orange juice

$1/2$ cup milk or soy milk

$1/2$ cup plain yogurt or soft tofu

1 tbsp flaxseed oil (optional)

1 tbsp flaxseeds (optional)

1. Place all ingredients in a blender, and blend for 1 minute or until smooth.

Makes 1 large or 2 medium shakes.

Variations: It's easy to adapt this recipe; if you prefer a thicker shake just add more banana or yogurt, or reduce the amount of milk. If you have some overripe peaches, use them instead of, or in addition to, the berries.

86

Nut Butter Smoothie

Start to finish time: 5 minutes

Prep time: 5 minutes

Unless allergies run in your family and you're avoiding nuts, this smoothie makes a delicious quick breakfast or snack. The molasses not only adds flavour and sweetness but also provides a hit of iron.

> 1 ripe banana
>
> 1 cup milk or soy milk
>
> $\frac{1}{2}$ cup yogurt
>
> 3 tbsp peanut, cashew, or almond butter
>
> 1 tbsp molasses (optional)
>
> $\frac{1}{4}$ tsp nutmeg (optional)
>
> 2 ice cubes

1. Place all ingredients in a blender, and blend for 1 minute or until smooth.

Makes 1 large or 2 medium shakes.

Variation: For a decadent peanut butter chocolate smoothie, add 1 tbsp each of cocoa powder and sugar.

87

15 minutes or less

Better than Basic Oatmeal

Start to finish time: 15 minutes

Prep time: 5 minutes

Cooking time: 10 minutes

Steel-cut oats are whole-grain groats that have been cut by steel discs. One cup contains more fibre than a bran muffin.

1 cup water

$^1/_2$ cup steel-cut oats

Optional add-ins:

$^1/_4$ cup fresh or frozen blueberries

2 tbsps chopped dried fruit such as raisins or figs

1 tbsp chopped nuts such as walnuts, hazelnuts, or almonds

1 tbsp whole or ground flaxseeds

$^1/_2$ tsp cinnamon

1. Place water and oats in a medium saucepan. Cover and soak overnight.
2. In the morning, bring the water and oats to a boil over medium-high heat. Reduce heat to low and simmer for 10 minutes (or according to the package's directions).
3. Add the optional add-ins of your choice. Serve with maple syrup or brown sugar, if desired.

Makes 1 serving.

Cottage Cheese Pancakes

Start to finish time: 15 minutes

Prep time: 5 minutes

Cooking time: 10 minutes

This recipe calls for dry cottage cheese, which can be found in plastic tubs or bags in the dairy section of the supermarket. If you can't find it, use ricotta that has been drained overnight in a paper towel–lined sieve set over a bowl in the refrigerator. Serve the pancakes with sliced fresh strawberries or banana, or with maple syrup.

3 eggs

1 tbsp canola oil

1 cup dry cottage cheese

$\frac{1}{4}$ cup all-purpose flour

$\frac{1}{4}$ tsp salt

1. Beat eggs lightly, and stir in oil and cottage cheese. Add flour and salt, and mix well.
2. Heat a lightly oiled frying pan over medium-high heat. Spoon about $\frac{1}{4}$ cup batter for each pancake into frying pan; cook for 1 $\frac{1}{2}$ to 2 minutes or until underside is golden. Flip and cook for 30 to 60 seconds longer, or until underside is golden. Repeat with remaining batter, brushing frying pan with more oil as necessary.

Makes 2 servings.

89

30
minutes
or less

Oatmeal Pancakes

Start to finish time: 30 minutes

Prep time: 10 minutes

Cooking time: 20 minutes

Pancakes are a wonderful weekend breakfast treat. These can be made ahead, frozen, and then reheated for days when you don't have time to stand over the stove. Leftovers make great cold snacks either plain or spread with low-fat cream cheese or peanut butter.

1 cup quick-cooking rolled oats

1 cup plain yogurt

1 cup 1% milk

1 tbsp packed brown sugar

1 tbsp butter

1 large egg, beaten

¼ cup canola oil

1 cup all-purpose flour

1 tbsp baking powder

1 tsp cinnamon

½ tsp salt

1. In a large bowl combine oats, yogurt, milk, and brown sugar and let sit for 5 minutes.
2. In a non-stick frying pan over medium heat, melt butter.
3. Whisk the egg and oil into the oat mixture.
4. In a medium bowl, combine the flour, baking powder, cinnamon, and salt. Add to the oat mixture and stir just until combined.

5. Spoon about ¼ cup batter for each pancake into frying pan; cook for 1 ½ to 2 minutes or until underside is golden brown and bubbles appear on top. Flip and cook for 30 to 60 seconds longer or until underside is golden brown. Repeat with remaining batter.

Makes 12 pancakes.

Make ahead: This recipe doubles well and freezes well. Stack each cooled pancake between sheets of waxed paper and wrap in plastic wrap. They'll keep for 2 to 3 months in the freezer. When you're ready to enjoy them, just peel pancakes from the waxed paper and reheat in the toaster oven, toaster, or microwave. You can also eat them cold.

Variation: If you don't have quick-cooking oats, substitute large-flake rolled oats and let the yogurt and milk mixture sit for 5 minutes longer.

Yogurt

Yogurt is an excellent source of protein and calcium. If possible choose yogurt labelled with "contains active cultures" or "living yogurt cultures" to get the benefits of probiotic bacteria, which help maintain a healthy intestinal tract and may protect against cancer and high cholesterol.

Eva's Energy Bars

Start to finish time: 30 minutes

Prep time: 10 minutes

Cooking time: 20 minutes, largely unattended

These are for mums who enjoy energy bars and are looking for an energy boost. (If you're not an energy bar fan, you'll probably prefer the Carrot Breakfast Bars on page 102.) Chopping sticky dried fruit like apricots can be time consuming, so check bulk food stores for prechopped dried fruit, or oil your knife before chopping.

3 cups large-flake rolled oats

1 cup all-purpose flour

1 cup packed brown sugar

1 cup chopped dried apricots

$\frac{2}{3}$ cup slivered almonds, toasted

$\frac{1}{2}$ cup wheat germ, toasted

$\frac{1}{2}$ cup golden raisins

2 eggs, beaten

$\frac{1}{2}$ cup canola oil

$\frac{1}{2}$ cup corn syrup

1. Preheat oven to 350°F. Line one 9- x 13-inch baking pan and one 8- x 8-inch baking pan with parchment paper.
2. In a large bowl combine oats, flour, brown sugar, apricots, almonds, wheat germ, and raisins.
3. In a small bowl, whisk together eggs, oil, and corn syrup. Add to oat mixture, stirring just until moistened.

92

4. Spread batter in prepared pans and bake for 20 to 25 minutes, until edges start to brown. Do not overcook. Let cool in baking pans until slightly warm, and cut into bars.

Makes 24 bars.

Make ahead: Store some of these bars in an airtight container and the rest, individually packaged in plastic wrap, in the freezer. They taste best defrosted, but I know mums who eat them straight from the freezer.

Lemon Blueberry Muffins

Start to finish time: 45 minutes

Prep time: 10 minutes

Cooking time: 35 minutes, largely unattended

These muffins were a mainstay of my diet after Madeleine was born. They are the easiest, fastest muffins I know, and who can resist the taste of tangy lemon mixed with antioxidant-laden blueberries? I ate them for breakfast and for snacks at home and on the run. This is one recipe where I don't recommend substituting whole wheat flour—it will make the muffins too heavy.

2 cups all-purpose flour

$^2/_3$ cup sugar

2 tsp baking powder

$^1/_2$ tsp baking soda

1 cup plain or vanilla yogurt

2 eggs, beaten

$^1/_3$ cup canola oil

Finely grated zest of 1 lemon

1 $^3/_4$ cups fresh or frozen blueberries

1. Preheat oven to 375°F. Line a 12-cup muffin tin with paper liners or grease lightly with oil or butter.
2. In a large bowl, combine flour, sugar, baking powder, and baking soda.
3. In a small bowl, whisk together yogurt, eggs, oil, and lemon zest. Stir into dry ingredients just until combined. Fold in blueberries.

4. Spoon batter into prepared muffin tin and bake for 35 minutes or until a toothpick inserted into muffin comes out clean. Let cool in pan for 5 minutes, then turn out muffins on rack and let cool completely.

Makes 12 muffins.

Make ahead: This recipe can easily be doubled. Store at room temperature up to 2 days, or freeze in resealable plastic bag or airtight container for up to 3 months.

Variation: For a banana and cinnamon variation, add 1 tsp ground cinnamon to the dry ingredients and omit the lemon zest. Replace the blueberries with 1 ¼ cups chopped bananas and ½ cup raisins.

Carrot Raisin Muffins

Start to finish time: 35 minutes

Prep time: 15 minutes

Cooking time: 20 minutes, largely unattended

You can make quick work of grating by using a food processor with a grater blade. Grating by hand doesn't take long either, and whichever you do, these muffins are worth the extra effort.

$\frac{1}{2}$ cup 1% milk

2 tbsp vinegar

$\frac{1}{4}$ cup All Bran™ cereal

1 $\frac{1}{4}$ cup all-purpose flour

$\frac{1}{2}$ cup packed brown sugar

1 $\frac{1}{2}$ tsp baking powder

$\frac{1}{2}$ tsp baking soda

$\frac{1}{2}$ tsp cinnamon

$\frac{1}{4}$ tsp nutmeg

1 cup grated carrots (approximately 2 large carrots)

$\frac{1}{2}$ cup raisins

1 egg, lightly beaten

$\frac{1}{3}$ cup canola oil

1. Preheat oven to 400°F. Line a 12-cup muffin tin with paper liners or grease lightly with oil or butter.
2. In a small bowl, combine milk and vinegar. Add the All Bran™, and let mixture sit for 5 minutes.

3. In a large bowl, combine flour, brown sugar, baking powder, baking soda, cinnamon, and nutmeg. Stir in the carrots and raisins.
4. Whisk together the egg and oil; add to the milk mixture. Pour over the flour mixture and stir just until combined.
5. Spoon batter into prepared muffin tin and bake for 20 minutes or until a toothpick inserted in a muffin comes out clean. Let cool in pan for 5 minutes, then turn out muffins on rack and let cool completely.

Makes 12 muffins.

Make ahead: This recipe can easily be doubled. Store at room temperature up for to 2 days, or freeze in resealable plastic bag or airtight container for up to 3 months.

Variation: If you don't have All Bran™ on hand, simply omit it, using 1 cup of all-purpose flour and ½ cup whole wheat flour instead.

Canola Oil

Neutral-flavoured canola oil is very low in saturated fat, relatively high in omega-3s and very high in monoun-saturated fat, which makes it beneficial for heart health and a great choice for baking.

97

Fruit Muffins

Start to finish time: 35 minutes

Prep time: 15 minutes

Cooking time: 20 minutes, largely unattended

These muffins were a hands-down favourite among my fellow-mum recipe testers. The dried fruit provides a welcome energy boost while the ginger adds lots of flavour.

1 $\frac{1}{2}$ cups whole wheat flour

$\frac{1}{2}$ cup large-flake rolled oats

$\frac{1}{3}$ cup sugar

2 tsp baking powder

1 tsp baking soda

2 eggs

$\frac{3}{4}$ cup plain or vanilla yogurt

$\frac{1}{3}$ cup canola oil

3 tbsp finely chopped crystallized ginger

1 cup finely chopped dried fruit (such as apricots, dates, and raisins)

1. Preheat oven to 400°F. Line a 12-cup muffin tin with paper liners or grease lightly with oil or butter.
2. In a medium bowl, combine flour, oats, sugar, baking powder, and baking soda.
3. In a large bowl, whisk together eggs, yogurt, oil, and ginger; stir in dried fruit. Pour over flour mixture and stir just until combined.

98

4. Spoon batter into prepared muffin tin and bake for 20 minutes or until toothpick inserted into muffin comes out clean. Let cool in pan for 5 minutes, then turn out muffins on rack and let cool completely.

Makes 12 muffins.

Paper Muffin Cups

Although it may seem less wasteful and more environmentally friendly to grease muffin tins, using paper liners instead will make cleanup quick and easy when time is at a premium.

Make ahead: This recipe can easily be doubled. Store at room temperature for up to 2 days, or wrap individually in plastic wrap and freeze in resealable plastic bag or airtight container for up to 3 months.

45
minutes
or less

Three-Grain Blueberry Muffins

Start to finish time: 40 minutes

Prep time: 15 minutes

Cooking time: 25 minutes, largely unattended

High in fibre and quick to prepare, these muffins can be thrown together once baby's down for her first nap of the day and before you shower. Pop the muffins into the oven and by the time you've showered, fresh, delicious muffins will await you.

1 cup 1% milk

$^1/_2$ cup quick-cooking rolled oats

$^3/_4$ cup all-purpose flour

$^1/_2$ cup cornmeal

$^1/_4$ cup wheat bran

1 tbsp baking powder

$^1/_4$ tsp salt

$^1/_3$ cup honey

$^1/_4$ cup canola oil

1 egg, beaten

Grated zest of one lemon

1 cup fresh or frozen blueberries

1. Preheat oven to 400°F. Line a 12-cup muffin tin with paper liners or grease lightly with oil or butter.
2. In a medium-sized, microwave-safe bowl, combine the milk and oats. Microwave on high until the oats are creamy and tender, 2 to 3 minutes.

3. Meanwhile, in a large bowl combine the flour, cornmeal, bran, baking powder, and salt.

4. To the milk and oat mixture, whisk in honey, oil, egg, and lemon zest. Pour over flour mixture and stir just until combined. Fold in blueberries.

5. Spoon batter into prepared muffin tin and bake for 20 minutes or until toothpick inserted into muffin comes out clean. Let cool in pan for 5 minutes, then turn out muffins on rack and let cool completely.

Makes 12 muffins.

Make ahead: This recipe can easily be doubled. Store at room temperature for up to 2 days, or wrap individually in plastic wrap and freeze in resealable plastic bag or airtight container for up to 3 months.

Using Soymilk in Baking

You can substitute vanilla soymilk for milk in most baking recipes, including breads, muffins, cakes, and cookies. Keep in mind that it tends to make baked goods appear darker.

Variation: You can replace the blueberries with raspberries and the lemon zest with the zest of 1 lime.

breakfasts and snacks

Carrot Breakfast Bars

Start to finish time: 55 minutes

Prep time: 25 minutes

Cooking time: 30 minutes, largely unattended

Although these bars may taste like cake, they're way better for you: they're loaded with vitamin-rich dried fruit, nuts, and carrots. Make these when you have a bit more time on your hands—they're not as fast to make as the muffins in this book.

1 ¹/₂ cups all-purpose flour

1 ¹/₂ cups whole wheat flour

2 tsp cinnamon

2 tsp baking powder

1 tsp baking soda

¹/₂ tsp ground ginger

¹/₄ tsp salt

2 eggs

1 cup mashed ripe bananas (2 large or 3 small)

³/₄ cup packed brown sugar

²/₃ cup plain or vanilla yogurt

¹/₃ cup canola oil

2 cups grated carrots (approximately 4 large carrots)

1 cup finely chopped dates or raisins

¹/₂ cup chopped pecans

1. Preheat oven to 375°F. Grease a 9- x 13-inch cake pan and line with parchment paper.

2. In a large bowl, combine all-purpose and whole wheat flours, cinnamon, baking powder, baking soda, ginger, and salt.
3. In a medium bowl, combine eggs, bananas, sugar, yogurt, and oil. Pour over flour mixture. Sprinkle with carrots, dates, and pecans, and stir just until combined.
4. Bake for 30 minutes or until toothpick inserted in centre comes out clean. Let cool in pan on rack before cutting into bars.

Makes 24 bars.

Make ahead: Store some of these bars in an airtight container for up to 3 days, and freeze the rest for up to 3 months. This recipe also doubles well.

Diane's Banana Bread

Start to finish time: 1 hour, 5 minutes

Prep time: 10 minutes

Cooking time: 55 minutes, largely unattended

Diane, a co-worker of mine and mother of one, kindly volunteered her foolproof banana bread recipe for this book. It was the snack of choice for both me and Madeleine after Lucy was born. Because bananas tend to turn brown quickly, it's useful to have recipes like this one to use them up. You can substitute chocolate chips for the raisins for a more decadent treat.

1 cup very ripe banana, mashed (approximately

    2 large or 3 small bananas)

²⁄₃ cup sugar

¹⁄₂ cup plain or vanilla yogurt

¹⁄₄ cup canola oil

2 eggs, beaten

1 ¹⁄₂ cups all-purpose flour

¹⁄₂ cup raisins

1 ¹⁄₂ tsp baking soda

1 tsp baking powder

¹⁄₂ tsp salt

1. Heat oven to 375°F. Lightly grease a 9- x 5-inch loaf pan.
2. In a large bowl, combine bananas, sugar, yogurt, oil, and eggs; mix thoroughly.
3. In a medium bowl, combine flour, raisins, baking soda,

baking powder, and salt. Add to banana mixture and stir
just until combined.

4. Pour batter into prepared pan. Bake 1 hour or until toothpick
   inserted into centre comes out clean. Let cool in pan 5 minutes before turning out onto a rack to cool completely.

Makes 1 loaf.

Make ahead: This recipe doubles
well to make 2 loaves. Wrap in
plastic wrap and store at room temperature for up to 2 days, or freeze
for up to 3 months.

Overripe Bananas

If you have over-
ripe bananas and
no time to bake,
peel them, wrap
them in plastic, and
store in the fridge
for up to 2 days or
in the freezer for
up to 2 months.

105

7

SMALL MEALS

15
minutes
or less

Garlicky Walnut Dip

Start to finish time: 5 minutes

Prep time: 5 minutes

Walnuts are a terrific source of omega-3 fatty acids, and they also contain iron, folate, and calcium. Buy them fresh from a bulk food store. Serve this dip with whole wheat pita, crackers, or veggies.

3 slices whole wheat bread

$^1/_4$ cup walnuts

3 cloves garlic, peeled

$^3/_4$ cup water

3 tbsp freshly squeezed lemon juice

1 tbsp virgin or extra-virgin olive oil

2 tbsp fresh parsley

Salt and freshly ground black pepper

1. Toast the bread and then process it in the food processor to fine crumbs.
2. With the food processor running, add the walnuts and garlic and process until finely ground.
3. With the food processor running, add the water, lemon juice, oil, parsley, salt, and pepper. Process until roughly the same consistency as hummus, adding more water if the mixture seems too dry.

Makes 1 $^1/_2$ cups.

108

Guacamole

15
minutes
or less

Start to finish time: 10 minutes

Prep time: 10 minutes

Avocados are full of healthy monounsaturated fats that are good for you and baby. Enjoy this guacamole as a dip with tortilla chips or raw veggies, a sandwich spread, or a condiment for tacos or quesadillas.

2 medium-ripe avocados

2 tbsp freshly squeezed lemon juice

1 medium-sized tomato, diced (optional, but really good)

$\frac{1}{4}$ cup plain yogurt

1–2 cloves garlic, minced

$\frac{1}{2}$ tsp salt

$\frac{1}{2}$ tsp cumin (optional)

$\frac{1}{2}$ tsp chili powder (optional)

$\frac{1}{4}$ tsp cayenne (optional)

1. Cut each avocado in half and remove pits. Scoop out flesh with a spoon and mash with a fork to desired consistency. Add lemon juice and mix.
2. Add tomato, yogurt, garlic, salt, cumin, chili powder, and cayenne, and mix well. Cover tightly and refrigerate for at least $\frac{1}{2}$ hour before eating.

Makes 2 cups.

109

Make ahead: Keeps in the fridge for up to 2 days, covered tightly with plastic wrap.

15
minutes
or less

Tina's Hummus

Start to finish time: 5 minutes with food processor,

10 minutes with blender

Prep time: 5 minutes

Tina and I met in a prenatal yoga class. Our due dates were one day apart and both our babies ended up coming two weeks late. She's also the source of the Lentil Soup recipe on page 160 and can be counted on to bring hummus and soup to every new mum she knows. Madeleine is so enamoured of her hummus that she won't accept any substitutes.

1 can (19 oz/540 mL) chickpeas

6 tbsp virgin or extra-virgin olive oil

4 tbsp freshly squeezed lemon juice

$^1\!/_4$ cup tahini

4 cloves garlic, peeled

1 $^1\!/_2$ tsp cumin

$^1\!/_2$ tsp salt

Cayenne to taste

$^1\!/_4$ cup water, approximately

1. Drain and rinse chickpeas, and place in the bowl of a food processor or in a blender. Add oil, lemon juice, tahini, garlic, cumin, salt, and cayenne, and process until smooth, adding water to reach desired consistency.

110 Makes 3 cups.

Variations: Have fun adapting this recipe to your taste. Add more garlic or cayenne if that's your style, or try a splash of hot pepper sauce. You can also substitute black beans for the chickpeas for a change.

Hummus

Hummus is amazingly versatile: it can be eaten as a dip with pita bread or veggies, used as a sandwich spread, or stuffed into a pita with cucumber, tomato, and lettuce. Although you can buy hummus ready-made in the supermarket, making it yourself is almost as quick and much cheaper.

Open-Face Sardine Sandwiches

Start to finish time: 5 minutes

Prep time: 5 minutes

Although you could just mash a tin of sardines onto some bread for a quick, nutritious lunch, if you've got a few extra minutes it's nice to gourmet it up a bit with this easy sandwich. You can substitute kippers for sardines.

1 can (3.75oz/106g) sardines, packed in water
2 slices whole-grain bread
1 tbsp finely chopped onion
1 tbsp plain yogurt
1 tsp Dijon mustard
$^{1}/_{2}$ tsp freshly squeezed lemon juice

1. Drain the sardines and mash them in a medium bowl.
2. Toast bread. Meanwhile, add onion, yogurt, mustard, and lemon juice to sardines and mix until thoroughly combined.
3. Divide sardine mixture between the 2 pieces of toast.

Makes 2 servings.

Guacamole, Tomato, and Brie Sandwich

15 minutes or less

Start to finish time: 5 minutes

Prep time: 5 minutes

After nine months plus of not eating brie cheese, now's the time to indulge a little. If you're short on time, skip making the guacamole and just use some slices of ripe avocado sprinkled with a little salt and freshly ground pepper—almost as tasty.

2 slices whole-grain bread

Guacamole (see recipe on page 109)

$^1/_2$ tomato, thinly sliced

4 oz brie, sliced

1. Toast bread, and spread one slice with guacamole. Top with tomato slices, brie, and remaining slice of bread.

Makes 1 serving.

15
minutes
or less

Justine's Basil, Tomato, and Avocado Sandwich

Start to finish time: 5 minutes

Prep time: 5 minutes

My sister-in-law, Justine, is a beleaguered vegetarian in a family of dedicated meat-eaters. However no one looks askance when she brings out these delicious sandwiches made with fresh-from-the-garden tomatoes. The piquant basil nicely offsets the mild flavour of the avocado. If you don't have fresh basil on hand, substitute pesto.

2 slices whole-grain bread

1 tsp Dijon mustard

$\frac{1}{2}$ tomato, thinly sliced

$\frac{1}{4}$ avocado, sliced

4 large basil leaves

Salt and freshly
    ground black pepper

1. Spread 1 slice of bread with Dijon mustard. Top with tomato, avocado, and basil, and sprinkle with salt and pepper. Top with remaining slice of bread.

Makes 1 serving.

Avocados

Avocados are high in fat, but most of that fat is heart-healthy mono- and polyunsaturated fat. They also contain vitamin E, folate, panthothenic acid, iron, zinc and fibre.

114

Salami, Pesto, Goat Cheese, and Tomato Sandwich

15 minutes or less

Start to finish time: 5 minutes

Prep time: 5 minutes

Every bite of this wonderful sandwich bursts with flavour. If you're on the move, pack the tomato separately and add it to the sandwich just before you eat it.

> 2 slices whole-grain bread or $\frac{1}{3}$ of a whole-grain baguette halved lengthwise
>
> 1 tsp Dijon mustard
>
> 2 tbsp goat cheese
>
> 2 tbsp pesto
>
> 6 slices of salami
>
> $\frac{1}{2}$ tomato thinly sliced

1. Spread one slice of bread with Dijon mustard; spread the other with goat cheese. Spread pesto on goat cheese, and top with salami, tomato, and remaining slice of bread.

Makes 1 serving.

small meals

Tuna Melts

Start to finish time: 10 minutes

Prep time: 5 minutes

Cooking time: 5 minutes

In this recipe the traditional mayonnaise is replaced with yogurt, making it a "light" lunch. The tuna mixture is also good cold in a pita pocket with cucumber and sprouts.

> 2–4 slices of bread (use 2 if you like a thick tuna melt; 4 for a thinner sandwich)
> 1 can (6.5 oz/184 g) light tuna in water, well drained
> 1 stalk celery, finely chopped
> 1 ½ tsp plain yogurt
> 1 tsp curry paste
> 1 clove garlic, minced
> ½ cup shredded Cheddar or Gouda

1. Turn oven to broil and toast bread on both sides.
2. Meanwhile, combine tuna, celery, yogurt, curry paste, and garlic, and mix well. Spread mixture on toasted bread and top with cheese. Broil until cheese is bubbly and tuna is heated through, 2 to 3 minutes. Serve immediately.

Makes 2 servings.

Variations: You can substitute green bell pepper for the celery in this recipe or add a chopped hard-boiled egg. You could also use canned salmon instead of tuna.

Tomato, Basil, and Feta Pasta

15 minutes or less

Start to finish time: 15 minutes

Prep time: 15 minutes

This makes a delicious lunch or light dinner, or even a side dish. Use the best tomatoes you can find, and if you don't have fresh basil, substitute ¹/₄ cup chopped parsley. You can increase the protein and fibre content of this dish by adding some cooked black beans. Other flavourful additions include pine nuts and chopped black olives.

16 oz small pasta shells

4 large or 5 medium tomatoes, chopped

6 tbsp olive oil

6 fresh basil leaves, finely sliced

1 clove garlic, minced

¹/₂ small red onion, finely chopped

Salt and freshly ground black pepper

1 ¹/₂ cups crumbled feta

2 tbsp grated Parmesan

1. In large pot of boiling salted water, cook pasta for 8 to 10 minutes or until tender but firm; drain well and return to pot.
2. Meanwhile, in a large bowl, combine tomatoes, oil, basil, garlic, and onion. Season with salt and pepper.
3. Toss hot cooked pasta with the tomato mixture, feta, and Parmesan. Serve warm or cold.

117

Makes 4 servings.

Almost Instant Pizza

Start to finish time: 20 minutes

Prep time: 5 minutes

Cooking time: 15 minutes, largely unattended

This is so easy to make for lunch or a light dinner, and you can use up whatever happens to be left in your refrigerator. My favourite combination is pesto, artichoke hearts, and goat cheese.

Large premade pizza crust

$^{1}/_{2}$ cup pizza sauce or pesto

Optional Toppings:

Anchovies, chopped

Artichoke hearts, drained and chopped

Bell peppers, seeded and sliced

Eggplant, thinly sliced

Feta, crumbled

Fresh basil

Goat cheese, crumbled

Lean ground beef, cooked

Lean ham, chopped

Mozzarella, grated

Mushrooms, sliced and sautéed

Olives

Pancetta, chopped

Prosciutto slices

Red onion, sliced

Steamed spinach

118

Tomato, sliced

Tuna, chopped

Zucchini, thinly sliced

1. Preheat oven to 350°F.
2. Top pizza crust with sauce or pesto and the toppings of your choice. Finish with mozzarella.
3. Bake for 10 to 15 minutes, until cheese is melted (or according to package directions for the crust).

Makes 2 servings.

Pancetta

Pancetta is an Italian bacon that is cured with salt and other spices but not smoked. Prosciutto or bacon can be substituted for pancetta in a pinch.

8

MAIN MEALS

Fried Rice with Eggs and Peas

15 minutes or less

Start to finish time: 15 minutes

Prep time: 5 minutes

Cooking time: 10 minutes

This recipe works best with precooked, cold rice, so make extra rice with your dinner the night before and you'll be able to whip up this dish in no time the next night.

4 tbsp canola oil

3 eggs, lightly beaten

3 cups cooked white rice, preferably cold

$\frac{1}{2}$ cup frozen peas, defrosted

1 tsp salt

$\frac{1}{2}$ cup green onion, finely sliced

Sweet chili sauce

1. Heat a wok or large frying pan over high heat. Add 2 tbsp of the oil and reduce heat to medium. Add eggs and allow to set for 20 seconds; scramble briefly. Transfer to a bowl.
2. Wipe the wok or frying pan with paper towel and return it to high heat. Add the 2 remaining tbsp of oil. Add rice and stir-fry for 2 minutes. If rice mixture appears dry, add a bit more oil.
3. Add peas and salt and stir-fry for another two minutes. Add the reserved eggs and the green onion and toss gently. Serve with sweet chili sauce on the side.

123

Makes 2 servings.

30 minutes or less

Salmon au Poivre

Start to finish time: 20 minutes

Prep time: 5 minutes

Cooking time: 15 minutes, largely unattended

This quick salmon dish is delicious, especially when you use the best and freshest salmon steaks you can find. Serve with basmati rice and steamed broccoli.

2 salmon steaks

Freshly ground black pepper

3 tbsp sherry or port

3 tbsp soy sauce

1 tbsp brown sugar

1. Preheat oven to 450°F. Rinse salmon and pat dry. Sprinkle both sides with black pepper.
2. In a shallow baking dish that will accommodate the salmon in a single layer, combine sherry, soy sauce, and brown sugar. Place salmon in the soy sauce mixture and turn to coat.
3. Bake salmon for 15 minutes or until fish flakes easily when tested with a fork.

Makes 2 servings.

Tip: This recipe is easy to adjust for more or fewer people. Just use 1 tbsp each of sherry and soy sauce and 1 tsp of brown sugar per steak, and add an extra tbsp each of sherry and soy sauce and an extra tsp of brown sugar to the total. So for 4 steaks you'd need 5 tbsp sherry, 5 tbsp soy sauce, and 5 tsp brown sugar.

Salmon

Salmon is an excellent source of omega-3s as well as vitamins B6 and B12, niacin and phosphorus. It's also low in saturated fat and cholesterol and a good source of protein. If possible choose wild salmon over farmed.

Salmon with Citrus Yogurt Sauce

Start to finish time: 25 minutes

Prep time: 10 minutes

Cooking time: 15 minutes

This tasty dish calls for Greek yogurt, which is thicker than regular yogurt and harder to find. If you don't have any luck tracking it down, you can substitute whole plain yogurt. If you have time, thicken the yogurt by putting it in a sieve lined with a double thickness of paper towel set over a bowl and letting it drain in the refrigerator for an hour or longer, discarding the liquid that drains off. Though this recipe calls for a salmon fillet, you can use salmon steaks if you prefer.

1 (1 lb) salmon fillet with skin, about 1 inch thick, deboned

$^3/_4$ tsp salt

$^1/_4$ tsp freshly ground black pepper

Citrus Yogurt Sauce:

1 cup low-fat plain Greek yogurt or plain whole-milk yogurt

2 tbsp olive oil

Grated zest of 1 lime

1 tbsp fresh lime juice

$^1/_2$ tsp grated orange zest

1 tsp orange juice

$^1/_2$ tsp salt

$^1/_2$ tsp honey

126

1. Preheat broiler. Line broiler pan or cookie tray with foil and lightly brush with olive oil.
2. Rinse fish, pat dry, place on broiler tray skin-side down, sprinkle with salt and pepper, and broil about 4 inches from heat for about 7 minutes. Tent fish with foil and continue broiling until cooked through, 7 to 9 minutes more, depending on your cut of salmon.
3. Citrus Yogurt Sauce: Meanwhile, in a small bowl combine yogurt, oil, lime zest and juice, orange zest and juice, salt, and honey. Serve salmon with sauce on the side.

Makes 4 servings.

Tip: If you have any Citrus Yogurt Sauce left over, it's delicious as a dip for strawberries.

127

30
minutes
or less

Broccoli and Anchovy Orecchiette

Start to finish time: 25 minutes

Prep time: 10 minutes

Cooking time: 15 minutes

If you can't find orecchiette, substitute penne rigate or fusilli in this recipe. Every ingredient, except for the broccoli and Parmesan, can be kept in the pantry and whipped up for a quick flavourful meal on the days you can't get to the grocery store. Make sure to buy broccoli that includes the stalk, not just the florets, for this dish, since the stalks are used to make the sauce.

2 large heads of broccoli, including stalks

1 lb orecchiette

$^1/_4$ cup extra-virgin olive oil

3–6 cloves garlic, peeled and chopped

8 anchovy fillets

2 small dried red chilies, crumbled

$^1/_4$ cup grated Parmesan

Salt and freshly ground black pepper

1. Remove the broccoli florets from the stalks and trim the dry ends off the stalks. Peel the stalks and finely chop them.
2. In a large pot of boiling salted water, cook pasta for 4 to 6 minutes or just until pasta is beginning to soften. Add broccoli florets and continue to cook for 4 minutes longer, until the pasta is tender but firm.

128

3. Meanwhile, in a large frying pan, heat oil over low heat. Add garlic, anchovies, and chilies; cover and cook for 8 to 10 minutes, or until the garlic is golden.
4. Drain pasta and broccoli well and add to anchovy mixture. Add the Parmesan, salt, and pepper, and toss well. Serve immediately.

Makes 4 servings.

Olive Oil

Olive oil is rich in monounsaturated fat, contains polyphenols, flavonoids and antioxidants, and has been linked with a reduced risk of heart disease and certain cancers. Rather than just adding olive oil to your diet, try replacing other fats, such as butter, with olive oil.

Asparagus or Broccoli Frittata

Start to finish time: 25 minutes

Prep time: 10 minutes

Cooking time: 15 minutes

Frittatas are almost as easy as omelettes but a little more elegant. Use asparagus in this recipe when it's in season and broccoli the rest of the time, or try using a mixture of the two.

1 tbsp olive oil

2 cups trimmed, chopped asparagus, or chopped broccoli florets

1 red bell pepper, seeded and diced

2 cloves garlic, minced

1 tsp dried thyme or 3 tsp chopped fresh thyme

$\frac{1}{2}$ tsp salt

$\frac{1}{4}$ tsp freshly ground black pepper

8 eggs

$\frac{1}{4}$ cup 1% milk

$\frac{1}{2}$ cup crumbled feta

1. Preheat broiler. In a 9-inch ovenproof frying pan (see tip on page 133), heat oil over medium-low heat. Cook asparagus, red pepper, garlic, thyme, salt, and pepper for 5 minutes, stirring occasionally, until the asparagus is just starting to get tender.

2. Meanwhile, in a large bowl, whisk eggs and milk. Add to the asparagus mixture and stir to combine. Reduce heat to low.

130

3. Sprinkle with feta and
   cook without stirring
   for 10 minutes, or until
   the edges are set but the
   centre is still soft. Broil
   for about 1 minute, or
   until the top is golden
   and set. Let sit for 5 minutes before sliding the
   frittata onto a plate.
   Cut into wedges and
   serve warm or at room
   temperature.

Makes 4 servings.

Broccoli

Broccoli, a seemingly
pedestrian veggie, is
laden with good things
like calcium, potassium,
folate, fibre, phytonutri-
ents, vitamins A and C
and even some iron. It's
also very versatile; try it
steamed, or in stir-fries,
pasta, and soups.

30
minutes
or less

Ham, Cheese, and Mushroom Frittata

Start to finish time: 25 minutes

Prep time: 10 minutes

Cooking time: 15 minutes

Feel free to add any leftover vegetables you happen to have in the refrigerator. Serve this frittata with some crusty whole-grain bread and salad or steamed vegetables to complete the meal.

2 tbsp olive oil

1 cup sliced mushrooms

$\frac{1}{2}$ medium onion, finely chopped

2 cloves garlic, minced

8 large eggs

1 $\frac{1}{3}$ cups chopped cooked ham

1 $\frac{1}{3}$ cups grated Cheddar

Salt and freshly ground black pepper

1. Preheat broiler. In a 9-inch ovenproof frying pan (see tip on page 133), heat 1 tbsp oil over medium-low heat. Add mushrooms, onion, and garlic, and cook 5 minutes or until onion is translucent and mushrooms start to brown.
2. Meanwhile, in a large bowl, whisk together eggs and stir in ham, half the Cheddar, and salt and pepper to taste.
3. Add the onion mixture to the egg mixture and combine well.
4. Add remaining 1 tbsp oil to frying pan and heat over low heat until hot but not smoking. Pour egg mixture into the

132

frying pan and distribute ingredients evenly. Cook without stirring for 10 minutes, or until the edges are set but the centre is still soft.

5. Sprinkle remaining cheese over the frittata and broil for 2 minutes or until the top is golden brown and set. Let sit for 5 minutes before sliding the frittata onto a plate. Cut into wedges and serve warm or at room temperature.

Makes 4 servings.

Make ahead: This frittata will keep in the refrigerator for up to 2 days, and in the freezer for up to 1 month.

Tip: If you don't have an ovenproof frying pan, you can use a regular frying pan and cover the handle with two layers of foil.

30 minutes or less

Beef Fajitas

Start to finish time: 25 minutes

Prep time: 10 minutes

Cooking time: 15 minutes

This easy dish is full of flavour and always a hit. Be sure to make extra so you'll have leftovers the next day.

1 tbsp chili powder

$^1/_2$ tsp ground oregano

$^1/_2$ tsp paprika

$^1/_4$ tsp cumin

$^1/_4$ tsp cayenne

$^1/_2$ tsp freshly ground black pepper

Pinch salt

$^1/_2$ pound beef sirloin, cut into $^1/_2$-inch strips

4 large whole wheat tortillas

1 tbsp olive oil

1 green, red, or yellow bell pepper, seeded and cut
  in strips

$^1/_2$ red onion, sliced

2 cloves garlic, crushed

2 cups shredded lettuce

1 medium tomato, diced

1 avocado diced, or Guacamole (see recipe on page 109)

$^1/_2$ cup shredded Cheddar

$^1/_2$ cup salsa

1. In a large resealable plastic bag, shake together the chili powder, oregano, paprika, cumin, cayenne, pepper, and salt. Add the beef and shake until well coated.
2. Heat tortillas according to package directions.
3. In a large non-stick frying pan, heat oil over medium heat. Add beef and cook for about 8 minutes or until browned but still pink inside. Add the bell pepper, onion, and garlic, and sauté until the vegetables are tender, about 5 minutes.
4. Assemble your fajitas by spooning beef into tortillas and topping with lettuce, tomato, avocado, Cheddar, and salsa. Roll up and serve.

Makes 4 servings.

30
minutes
or less

Shrimp, Veggie, and Cashew Stir-Fry

Start to finish time: 30 minutes

Prep time: 15 minutes

Cooking time: 15 minutes

You can use any combination of fish, vegetables, and nuts in this recipe. Try asparagus instead of broccoli, halibut instead of shrimp, and almonds instead of cashews.

1 ½ cups rice

1 ½ cups baby spinach, rinsed and drained

2 tbsp soy sauce

1 tbsp red wine vinegar

1 tsp minced fresh gingerroot

1 clove garlic, finely chopped

2 cups broccoli florets

2 yellow or red bell peppers, seeded and sliced in strips

2 green onions, cut in 1-inch pieces

3 tbsp canola oil

1 tbsp sesame oil

1 lb large, raw shrimp, fresh or frozen, peeled

½ cup cashews, whole or pieces

1. Cook rice according to package directions.
2. Heat a wok or large frying pan over medium heat. Add spinach, cover, and steam until wilted, 3 to 4 minutes. Remove spinach, squeeze dry, and set aside.

136

3. In a medium bowl combine soy sauce, gingerroot, vinegar, and garlic. Add the broccoli, bell peppers, and green onions and mix well.

4. In the wok or frying pan, heat canola oil and sesame oil over medium-high heat. Add the vegetable mixture and stir-fry for 3 to 5 minutes, until vegetables are crisp-tender. Add shrimp and cook an additional 4 to 5 minutes, until shrimp are pink.

5. In individual bowls layer spinach over rice, then top with the shrimp mixture and a sprinkle of cashews.

Makes 4 servings.

Tip: Frozen shrimp do not need to be fully defrosted before cooking, but they'll cook faster if you rinse them under hot water before adding them to the pan.

Cashews

Cashews are lower in total fat than most nuts but higher in saturated fat. Still, they are a good source of protein and unsaturated fatty acids, and they contain the B vitamins thiamin, riboflavin, niacin, and B6, as well as iron, magnesium, vitamin E, folate and calcium.

137

Chicken and Black Bean Quesadillas

Start to finish time: 30 minutes

Prep time: 20 minutes

Cooking time: 10 minutes

Baking these quesadillas rather than frying them will require less of your undivided attention. Serve them with Guacamole (see recipe on page 109) or chopped avocado, chopped tomatoes, and sour cream or yogurt. If you have any left over, have them for lunch the next day. Just reheat them in foil or in the microwave so the tortilla doesn't get too crunchy.

2 $^1/_2$ cups shredded chicken*

1 cup canned black beans, rinsed and drained

1 tsp chili powder

1 tsp salt

$^1/_2$ tsp freshly ground black pepper

$^1/_2$ tsp cumin

$^1/_2$ large onion, thinly sliced

3 garlic cloves, thinly sliced

1 cup grated Monterey Jack cheese

2 whole wheat tortillas

* Use leftover chicken or precooked rotisserie chicken.

1. Preheat oven to 400°F.
2. In a large bowl, combine chicken, black beans, $^1/_2$ tsp chili powder, $^1/_2$ tsp salt, $^1/_4$ tsp pepper, and $^1/_4$ tsp cumin.

3. In a small frying pan over medium heat, sauté onion with remaining $\frac{1}{2}$ tsp chili powder, $\frac{1}{2}$ tsp salt, $\frac{1}{4}$ tsp pepper, and $\frac{1}{4}$ tsp cumin for about 6 minutes, or until golden. Add garlic and cook, stirring, until fragrant. Add to chicken mixture along with cheese, and toss until well combined.
4. Spread about $\frac{1}{2}$ cup of the chicken mixture onto half of each tortilla, fold over and place on 9- x 13-inch nonstick baking sheet. Bake for about 10 minutes, or until heated through. Flip quesadillas halfway through baking.

Makes 4 servings.

Variation: Instead of using black beans, substitute 1 cup of canned chickpeas blended with 1 tbsp olive oil in a blender or food processor.

Chicken, Bean, and Spinach Soup

Start to finish time: 35 minutes

Prep time: 15 minutes

Cooking time: 20 minutes, largely unattended

This hearty soup is full of protein and fibre and low in fat. Save time by getting your butcher to chop the chicken for you and by buying prewashed baby spinach.

1 tbsp olive oil

2 cloves garlic, minced

1 tbsp minced fresh gingerroot

2 skinless, boneless chicken breasts, chopped in
  1-inch pieces

2 carrots, peeled and sliced

1 sweet potato, peeled and diced in 1-inch pieces

1 can (10 oz/284 ml) low-sodium chicken broth,
undiluted

1 can (10 oz/284 ml) water

3 ½ cups baby spinach

1 can (19 oz/540 ml) romano, kidney, or garbanzo
  (chickpeas) beans, drained and rinsed

½ tsp freshly ground black pepper

1. In large saucepan, heat oil over medium-high heat. Add garlic and gingerroot, and sauté for 1 minute. Add chicken and sauté until no longer pink. Add carrots, sweet potato, chicken broth, and water, and bring to a boil. Reduce heat,

cover, and simmer for 20 minutes, or until carrots and sweet potato are tender.

2. Stir in spinach, beans, and pepper. Heat through and serve.

Makes 4 servings.

Make ahead: This soup will keep in an airtight container for up to 3 days in the refrigerator and up to 4 months in the freezer.

Sweet Potatoes

Sweet potatoes are high in beta carotene, which may help slow the aging process and reduce the risk of some cancers, and they're a good source of fibre, vitamins B-6, C and E, folate, and potassium. Eat them with their skins on if possible, as that's where much of their benefits lie.

141

Pollo Salsa Verde

Start to finish time: 35 minutes

Prep time: 15 minutes

Cooking time: 20 minutes, largely unattended

Pollo Salsa Verde means "Green Salsa Chicken." Salsa verde is made with tomatillos rather than the more traditional tomatoes. If you can't find it in your grocery store, you may need to seek out a deli or a store specializing in Mexican products. When you do find it, stock up.

1 ¹/₂ cups rice

1 tbsp olive oil

2 boneless, skinless chicken breasts cut in 1-inch pieces

2 cans (each 19 oz/540 ml) white kidney or white navy
   beans, drained and rinsed

1 ¹/₂ cups green salsa (salsa verde)

1 large tomato, diced

¹/₄ cup chopped cilantro

¹/₂ cup grated Monterey Jack cheese

1. Cook rice according to package directions.
2. In a large saucepan, heat oil over medium heat. Add
   chicken and sauté until no longer pink, about 5 minutes.
3. Add beans, salsa, tomato, and cilantro; bring to
   a boil. Reduce heat to a simmer and cook for 15 minutes.
   Serve the chicken over rice, sprinkled with Monterey Jack.

142

Makes 4 servings.

Make ahead: This recipe can be doubled and even tripled. It will keep in an airtight container in the refrigerator for up to 4 days, or in the freezer for up to 3 months.

Ice Cube Trays

Ice cube trays are handy tools to have in your kitchen. Use them to freeze cubes of leftover broth, milk, juice, tomato paste, pesto, and even wine for future cooking. Once baby starts eating solids, you can use the trays to freeze baby food as well.

White Chili

Start to finish time: 50 minutes

Prep time: 20 minutes

Cooking time: 30 minutes, largely unattended

This "white" version of chili combines chicken and chickpeas for a tasty, unfussy dinner. It can be left to simmer anywhere from 20 minutes to an hour, so you can be there for your baby when he hasn't settled down to sleep or has begun a marathon nursing session. In fact, the longer the chili cooks, the better it tastes.

2 tsp canola oil

1 cup diced onion

2 cups sliced mushrooms

1 cup diced green bell pepper

1 cup diced carrots

4 cloves garlic, minced

12 oz boneless, skinless chicken breasts (about 3 breasts), cut in 1-inch pieces

$\frac{1}{4}$ cup cornstarch

1 can (23 oz/680 ml) plain tomato sauce

1 can (19 oz/540 ml) white chickpeas, drained and rinsed

1 cup low-sodium chicken stock

1 tbsp fresh basil, shredded

2 tsp chili powder

1 tsp dried oregano

1 tsp ground cumin

Cayenne pepper

$\frac{1}{3}$ cup chopped fresh cilantro or parsley

6 tbsp shredded Monterey Jack cheese

1. In a large non-stick frying pan, heat oil over medium heat. Add onion and sauté for 5 minutes or until golden. Stir in mushrooms, green pepper, carrots, and garlic, and cook, stirring frequently, for 10 minutes, or until vegetables begin to soften and mushrooms have begun to brown.
2. Put chicken and cornstarch in a large plastic bag, close, and shake until chicken is coated (this will keep it moist). Add chicken to vegetables and cook for 5 minutes, stirring constantly, or until chicken is no longer pink inside.
3. Add tomato sauce, chickpeas, chicken stock, basil, chili powder, oregano, cumin, and cayenne pepper to taste, and bring to boil. Reduce heat, cover, and simmer for at least 20 minutes and for up to an hour. (The longer it simmers, the better it tastes.)
4. Serve sprinkled with Monterey Jack and fresh cilantro.

Makes 4 to 6 servings.

Make ahead: This recipe doubles well and will keep in an airtight container in the refrigerator for up to 4 days, or in the freezer for up to 3 months.

AJ's Whole Wheat Mac 'n' Cheese

Start to finish time: 50 minutes

Prep time: 20 minutes

Cooking time: 30 minutes, largely unattended

Yes, you could just make the boxed variety of mac 'n' cheese, but this homemade version is a cut above in taste and nutrition. And making it doesn't take much more effort. Make big batches and freeze in dinner-sized portions so you have a quick, easy meal available.

2 cups whole wheat macaroni

3 tsp butter

1 medium onion, diced

⅓ cup all-purpose flour

3 cups 2% milk

2 cups grated Cheddar

1 tbsp Dijon mustard

2 slices of whole wheat bread

2 tbsp Parmesan (optional)

1. In a large pot of boiling salted water, cook macaroni for 8 to 10 minutes or until tender but firm; drain well and return to pot.

2. Meanwhile, preheat oven to 350°F. Butter a 9- x 13-inch casserole dish.

3. In a large saucepan, melt 2 tsp of the butter over medium-high heat. Add onion and sauté about 4 minutes, or until softened. Sprinkle flour over onion and cook, stirring for

146

30 seconds, or until flour is lightly browned. Whisk in milk. Bring to a boil and cook for 5 minutes.

4. Remove from the heat and add the Cheddar and mustard, and stir until smooth.

5. Add the cooked macaroni to the cheese sauce, stirring to combine. Spoon the mixture into the prepared casserole dish.

6. Place bread in the bowl of a food processor, and process until fine crumbs.

7. In a small saucepan melt the remaining 1 tsp of butter and add it to the bread crumbs along with the Parmesan if using. Toss mixture together and sprinkle over macaroni.

8. Bake uncovered for 30 to 40 minutes. (For the batches you're going to freeze, skip this step, and just thaw and cook before serving.)

Makes 4 servings.

Make ahead: This recipe doubles well. Prepare it through Step 7, then store tightly wrapped in the fridge for up to 3 days and in the freezer for up to 3 months.

Variations: If you have some leftover ham, add 1 cup of diced ham, along with the Cheddar in Step 4. You can also add 1 cup of frozen peas along with the Cheddar in Step 4.

147

Easy Baked Penne

Start to finish time: 55 minutes

Prep time: 25 minutes

Cooking time: 30 minutes, largely unattended

Dubbed "Lazy Lasagna" by testers, this pasta dish is vegetarian and is loaded with fresh vegetables.

4 cups penne

1 tbsp olive oil

2 cups chopped broccoli

1 cup sliced carrots

1 cup seeded and chopped green bell pepper

$^1/_2$ cup sliced mushrooms

4 cloves garlic, minced

4 large or 5 medium tomatoes, chopped

2 tbsp fresh basil, shredded, or 2 tsp dried basil

2 tsp dried oregano

1 tsp freshly ground black pepper

1 $^1/_2$ cups grated mozzarella

1 cup Parmesan

1. Preheat oven to 375°F. Lightly butter a 9- x 13-inch baking dish.
2. In a large pot of boiling salted water, cook pasta for 8 to 10 minutes, or until tender. Drain well and return to pot.
3. Meanwhile, in a large non-stick frying pan, heat oil over medium heat. Add broccoli, carrots, and green bell pepper and sauté until tender, about 5 minutes. Add mushrooms and garlic, and cook for another 5 minutes.

4. Add the tomatoes, basil, oregano, and pepper to the vegetable mixture, and reduce heat to low. Simmer for 3 to 5 minutes.

5. Transfer the vegetable mixture to a large bowl, add the cooked, drained pasta and 1 cup of the mozzarella; toss gently to mix. Spoon pasta mixture into prepared dish, and sprinkle with Parmesan and remaining mozzarella. Cover the baking dish with a lid or foil, and bake for 15 minutes. Remove cover and bake another 15 minutes, or until golden and bubbly.

Makes 4 servings.

Make ahead: This recipe can be prepared the night before and popped into the oven for dinner the next day. It can easily be doubled and will keep, covered tightly, in the refrigerator for up to 3 days, or in the freezer for up to 3 months.

Even Easier Baked Penne

Start to finish time: 40 minutes

Prep time: 10 minutes

Cooking time: 30 minutes, largely unattended

If you've got your pantry well stocked you can make this dinner without a single trip to the store. If you do have fresh produce on hand, then serve this with a salad or some steamed broccoli to complete the meal.

3 cups penne

25 oz marinara pasta sauce of your choice, or 3 cups
Andrew's Spaghetti Sauce (see recipe on page 156)

1 cup ricotta

1 tbsp fresh basil, shredded, or 1 tsp dried basil

Salt and freshly ground black pepper

1 $^1/_2$ cup mozzarella, grated

1. Preheat the oven to 350°F. Lightly butter a 9- x 9-inch baking dish.
2. In a large pot of boiling salted water, cook pasta for 8 to 10 minutes, or until tender but firm. Drain well and return to pot for 5 minutes.
3. Meanwhile, in a large bowl, combine 2 cups pasta sauce, ricotta, and basil; season with salt and pepper.
4. Add the cooked, drained pasta to the pasta sauce mixture and toss gently to combine. Spread $^1/_2$ cup of the remaining pasta sauce on the bottom of the baking dish. Spoon the pasta mixture into the baking dish and drizzle the

150

remaining ¹/₂ cup pasta sauce over top. Sprinkle with mozzarella.

5. Cover baking dish with lid or foil and bake for 15 minutes. Remove cover and bake for another 15 minutes, or until golden and bubbly.

Makes 4 servings.

Make ahead: This recipe doubles well and can be stored, tightly covered, in the refrigerator for up to 3 days or in the freezer for up to 3 months.

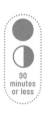

90
minutes
or less

One-Hour Oven Chicken Dinner

Start to finish time: 1 hour, 15 minutes

Prep time: 15 minutes

Cooking time: 1 hour, largely unattended

Though this meal has to cook for about an hour, it can be assembled in a few minutes, leaving you time to sort the laundry, empty the dishwasher, sweep up the dust bunnies, take your baby to the park, return phone calls, or just sit with your baby and watch the world go by.

2 tbsp unsalted butter

8 boneless, skinless chicken thighs, rinsed and patted dry

1/2 cup soy sauce

1/2 cup dry sherry

2 cloves garlic, chopped

1 tbsp grated gingerroot

2 tsp packed brown sugar

3 medium sweet potatoes, unpeeled and halved
   lengthwise

1 cup rice

2 cups water or low-sodium chicken stock

1/4 cup frozen peas

1 tbsp sesame seeds (optional)

1 small head broccoli, cut in florets

1. Preheat oven to 350°F. Put butter in a 9- x 11-inch baking pan and place in oven until butter is melted.

2. Meanwhile, in a 9- x 13-inch casserole dish, combine soy sauce, sherry, garlic, and gingeroot. Add chicken thighs in a single layer and turn to coat. Cover with lid or foil.

3. Remove baking pan from oven and add brown sugar, stirring to combine. Arrange sweet potatoes in pan in a single layer, cut side down.

4. Rinse rice and put it in a small casserole dish. Add water and peas. Cover with lid or foil.

5. Put chicken dish, rice dish, and sweet potatoes in the oven and bake for 50 minutes. Turn chicken and sprinkle with sesame seeds. Bake everything 10 minutes longer.

6. Steam broccoli while the chicken finishes cooking.

Makes 4 servings.

Tip: Make extra rice with this dinner and use it to make Fried Rice with Eggs and Peas (see recipe on page 123) the next night.

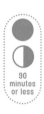

Salmon and Spinach Quiche

Start to finish time: 1 hour, 20 minutes

Prep time: 20 minutes

Cooking time: 1 hour

This recipe is so easy, so fast to prepare, and so delicious that it's a staple at our house. We make it with the hope that the goodness of the salmon, eggs and spinach works to offset the less salubrious effects of the cream and pie crust. We never make less than two at a time, which is why this recipe makes two quiches, and often we'll make four. Leftovers are great for lunch or even breakfast. This recipe makes two quiches, because you might as well make two while baby is down for her afternoon nap: one for dinner and one for the freezer.

2 9-inch pastry shells

4 large eggs

2 cups half-and-half cream

Freshly ground black pepper

2 cans (7.5 oz/222 mL each) boneless, skinless wild
   salmon, drained

2 cups grated Cheddar

2 cups chopped baby spinach

10 leaves fresh basil, shredded

$^1/_4$ cup grated Parmesan (optional)

1. Preheat oven to 375°F. Bake pastry shells for 10 minutes. Remove from oven and reduce temperature to 350°F.
2. Meanwhile, whisk together the eggs, cream, and pepper.

154

3. In each pastry shell, layer 1 can of salmon, 1 cup of Cheddar, 1 cup of spinach, and half the basil. Pour half the egg mixture over each shell and sprinkle with Parmesan, if using. Bake for 55 to 65 minutes. Let sit for 5 minutes before serving.

Makes 6 to 8 servings.

Make ahead: This recipe can easily be doubled. It will keep, tightly wrapped, in the refrigerator for up to 2 days and in the freezer for up to 1 month.

Eggs

Eggs, it seems, may have gotten a bad rap. Recent research shows that our total and saturated fat intake has more effect on our cholesterol levels than dietary cholesterol. Eggs are a great source of protein and contain vitamin B12, riboflavin, vitamin D, folate and iron.

Andrew's Spaghetti Sauce

Start to finish time: 1 hour, 20 minutes

Prep time: 20 minutes

ng time: 1 hour or more, largely unattended

My husband, Andrew, who's a willing but inexperienced cook, is (justifiably) proud of this spaghetti sauce, which he's perfected over the years. Every couple of weekends he makes a big batch of it, and we use it to make everything from lasagna to Even Easier Baked Penne (see recipe on page 150).

1 tbsp olive oil

3 large carrots, sliced

3 stalks celery, sliced

$1/2$ small onion, finely chopped

3.5 oz (approx.) pancetta

4 cloves garlic, minced

1 lb extra-lean ground beef

6–10 mushrooms, sliced

$1/2$ cup red wine (optional)

3 cans (each 23 oz/680 ml) plain tomato sauce

2 tsp Worcestershire sauce

10 leaves fresh basil, shredded, or 2 tsp dried basil

2 tsp oregano

1 tsp sage

1 tsp cayenne

2 bay leaves

Salt and freshly ground black pepper

156

1. In a large pot, heat oil over medium-high heat. Add carrots, celery, onion, pancetta, and garlic, and cook for 10 minutes or until vegetables have softened. Remove vegetables and set aside.
2. Return pot to medium-high heat, and add ground beef. Cook, stirring occasionally, until browned. Drain fat, and add mushrooms and wine, if using; cook for another 5 minutes, stirring occasionally, until wine evaporates a little.
3. Add reserved cooked vegetables, tomato sauce, Worcestershire sauce, basil, oregano, sage, cayenne, bay leaves, salt, and pepper; bring to a boil, reduce heat, and simmer, uncovered, for at least an hour, stirring occasionally.

Makes 6 to 8 servings.

Make ahead: This recipe doubles well, and will keep in an airtight container in the refrigerator for up to 3 days and in the freezer for up to 3 months.

Fresh Herbs

Some herbs—basil, for example—are so much better fresh that it seems a shame to use dried. If a recipe calls for a dried herb, you can substitute fresh but use three times the amount of the dried called for. For example, instead of adding 1 tsp of dried basil or thyme, add 1 tbsp of fresh.

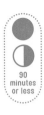

Garlic Ginger Sweet Potato Soup

Start to finish time: 1 hour, 25 minutes

Prep time: 25 minutes

Cooking time: 1 hour, largely unattended

This is a nice twist on the ubiquitous carrot ginger soup. This recipe makes a huge batch, but it freezes well and having some on hand can be a lifesaver when you simply don't have the time or energy to cook.

1 tbsp canola oil

6 large sweet potatoes, halved lengthwise

7 cloves garlic, unpeeled

3 slices peeled gingerroot

6 cups chicken broth, low sodium if possible

1 to 2 cups water

1. Preheat oven to 350°F. Pour oil on baking sheet and heat until hot.
2. Rub cut sides of sweet potatoes in the warm oil and place cut side down on baking sheet. Scatter garlic and gingerroot over sweet potatoes and bake, uncovered, 45 to 60 minutes, or until potatoes are soft.
3. Scoop pulp from potato skins and place in bowl of food processor or blender. Squeeze garlic from skins and add to sweet potato pulp. Add gingerroot to sweet potato and process, adding chicken broth as needed to make a purée. Depending on the size of your food processor or blender, it may be easier to do this in batches.

158

4. Pour sweet potato puree into a large saucepan. Add remaining broth and as much water as needed to reach desired consistency; cook over medium-low heat until heated through, stirring frequently to prevent soup sticking to the bottom of pot. Serve with a dollop of sour cream or yogurt on top.

Makes 8 servings.

Make ahead: This soup will keep in an airtight container in the refrigerator for up to 3 days and in the freezer for up to 4 months.

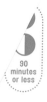

Lentil Soup

Start to finish time: 1 hour, 30 minutes

Prep time: 20 minutes

Cooking time: 1 to 2 hours, largely unattended

Lentils are rich in dietary fibre and an excellent source of B vitamins and protein. They also readily absorb myriad flavours and, compared with other dried legumes, are relatively quick and easy to prepare. This soup is just one way to enjoy lentils, and it may well become a new mum's favourite. Served with some crusty whole-grain bread, it's a hearty meal all on its own.

1 ½ cups lentils, rinsed

6 cups water

1 tsp salt

3 medium potatoes, peeled and chopped

2 cups chopped celery

1 large onion, finely chopped

1 green bell pepper, seeded and diced

1 cup sliced carrots

1 can (28 oz/796 mL) diced or crushed tomatoes

2 cloves garlic

2 tbsp olive oil

1 bay leaf

Salt and freshly ground black pepper

Red wine vinegar or balsamic vinegar (optional)

1. In a large soup pot, combine lentils, water, and salt over high heat. Bring to a boil, reduce heat, and simmer for 20 minutes while you wash and chop the vegetables.

2. Add potatoes, celery, onion, green pepper, carrots, tomatoes, garlic, olive oil, bay leaf, salt, and black pepper to taste to the lentils. Bring to a boil, reduce heat, and simmer, uncovered, stirring occasionally, for 1 to 2 hours. If soup starts to get too thick, add more water.

3. Adjust seasonings to taste and serve soup hot, drizzled with some red wine or balsamic vinegar.

Makes 8 servings.

Make ahead: This will keep in an airtight container in the refrigerator for up to 3 days or in the freezer for up to 4 months.

Lentils

Lentils are low in fat and calories, high in protein, fibre and folate, and they're also a source of iron, phosphorus, zinc, and magnesium. Lentils are the quickest legume to cook and can be used in salads, soups, stews, and rice.

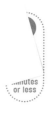

Beef Stew

...minutes
or less

Start to finish time: 2 hours

Prep time: 20 minutes

Cooking time: 1 to 1 ½ hours, largely unattended

This stew takes a long time to cook, but once it's simmering it doesn't need your attention until you're ready to eat. It's a wholesome, delicious meal for cold winter nights. Serve it with a crusty loaf of whole-grain bread and a salad if you're feeling ambitious. This recipe should make enough for a couple of dinners, which is always a bonus.

2 tbsp olive oil

2 medium onions, roughly chopped

2 tbsp all-purpose flour

3 cups chicken, beef, or vegetable stock

2–2 ½ lbs lean stewing beef cut in 1-inch pieces

¼ cup pearl barley, rinsed

1 bay leaf

1 tsp fresh thyme leaves or ⅓ tsp dried thyme

4 large or 5 medium potatoes, peeled and cut in 1-inch chunks

4 large carrots, peeled and sliced

2 leeks, rinsed and chopped, whites only (optional)

8 cloves garlic, peeled (optional)

1 cup fresh or frozen peas

1 clove garlic, minced

Salt and freshly ground black pepper

1. In a large heavy pot, heat oil over medium-high heat. Add onion and cook, stirring frequently, for 7 minutes or until they soften. Sprinkle flour over the onion and cook, stirring, for 2 minutes or until the flour is lightly browned.
2. Add the stock, stirring to combine. Add beef, barley, bay leaf, and thyme, and bring to a boil. Reduce heat, cover and simmer for 30 minutes. The stew should still be quite thin; if not, add more stock or water.
3. Meanwhile, chop the remaining vegetables. Add the potatoes, carrots, leeks, and garlic if using, and bring back to a boil. Lower the heat, cover and simmer for 30 to 60 minutes or until the meat and vegetables are tender.
4. Add the peas and minced garlic and simmer, uncovered, for a few minutes until the flavour of the garlic has permeated the stew and the peas are warm. Season with salt and pepper to taste.

Makes 6 to 8 servings.

Make ahead: This recipe can easily be doubled and will keep in an airtight container in the refrigerator for up to 4 days or in the freezer for up to 3 months.

ACKNOWLEDGEMENTS

If it takes a village to raise a child, then it takes a metropolis to write a book while you're raising one child and pregnant with another. There are so many people without whom this book would never have been written: my husband, Andrew, who took up all the slack—and there was a lot of it; my mum, Anne, a writer herself, who not only helped me get this project off the ground but had a standing play date with Madeleine; my dad, Dirk, who took on chauffeur duties; my sister, Nadaleen, for being the best Auntie Nanny; my editors Tanya Trafford and Stacey Cameron—Tanya for believing in the idea in the first place and Stacey for making sure it made it all the way to the finish line; all my friends who contributed stories, recipes, ideas, and support, and who tested recipes and let me talk, thanks to Andrea, Angela, Ann, Anne, Becky, Chantelle, Ellen, Emma, Gwen, Heidi, Helen, Janet, Julie, Justine, Kylie, Megan, Melodie, Naomi, Tanya, Tiffany, Tina, and Victoria; Gramma B and Grampa Dave for Nanaimo weekends; and to Laurie Bailey,

Margot Davidson, Noony Paletta, and Diana Steele for their expertise and for letting me pick their brains. And finally thank you to Madeleine and Lucy—this book would never have been written if you hadn't slept so well!

healthy mum, happy baby

APPENDIX A: MORE INFORMATION
ON BREASTFEEDING

Reading

The Breastfeeding Book by Dr. William Sears

Dr. Jack Newman's Guide to Breastfeeding by Jack Newman
and Teresa Pitman

Surfing

Canadian Breastfeeding Foundation
   http://www.canadianbreastfeedingfoundation.org
Canadian Pediatric Society: Breastfeeding
   http://www.caringforkids.cps.ca/babies/Breastfeeding.htm
INFACT Canada
   http://www.infactcanada.ca/InfactHomePage.htm
La Leche League Canada
   http://www.lalecheleaguecanada.ca
La Leche League International
   http://www.lalecheleague.org

167

Mayo Clinic: Baby Feeding

http://www.mayoclinic.com/health/healthy-baby/FL00111

Motherisk

http://www.motherisk.org/women/index.jsp (This site gives information on the safety of drugs, chemicals and disease during pregnancy and lactation.)

ProMom

http://www.promom.org

(This site promotes public awareness and acceptance of breastfeeding.)

World Health Organization, Global Strategy for Infant and Young Child Feeding

http://www.who.int/child-adolescent-health/NUTRITION/global_strategy.htm

healthy mum, happy baby

APPENDIX B: MORE INFORMATION ON DIET AND NUTRITION

Reading

Child of Mine: Feeding with Love and Good Sense by Ellyn Satter

Leslie Beck's Nutrition Guide to a Healthy Pregnancy: What to Eat Before, During, and After Your Pregnancy by Leslie Beck

Mealtime Solutions for Your Baby, Toddler and Preschooler by Ann Douglas

Secrets of Feeding a Healthy Family by Ellyn Satter

What to Eat Before, During, and After Pregnancy by Judith E. Brown

Surfing

3-A-Day of Dairy
http://www.3aday.org/3aDay

5 to 10 a Day for Better Health
http://www.5to10aday.com

Canada's Food Guide to Healthy Eating
http://www.hc-sc.gc.ca/fn-an/
food-guide-aliment/index_e.html

Dietitians of Canada
http://www.dietitians.ca/

Food News From the Environmental Working Group
http://www.foodnews.org

Health Canada: Children and Healthy Eating
http://www.hc-sc.gc.ca/fn-an/nutrition/child-enfant/
index_e.html

Health Canada: Infant Feeding
http://www.hc-sc.gc.ca/fn-an/nutrition/child-enfant/
infant-nourisson/index_e.html

Healthy Mom: Essential Fats Information for Moms
http://www.vitalchoice.com/healthymom/index.cfm

Heart & Stroke Foundation: Healthy Eating
http://ww2.heartandstroke.ca/Page.asp?PageID=
38&SubCategoryID=128&Src=living&Type=Article

Mayo Clinic: Food & Nutrition
http://www.mayoclinic.com/health/food-and-nutrition/
NU99999

Nutrition for Healthy Term Infants: A joint statement by
the Canadian Paediatric Society, Health Canada, and
Dietitians of Canada
http://www.hc-sc.gc.ca/fn-an/pubs/infant-nourrisson/
nut_infant_nourrisson_term_e.html

APPENDIX C: MORE
QUICK AND EASY RECIPES

Reading

How to Cook Everything by Mark Bittman
The Instant Cook by Donna Hay
Life's on Fire: Cooking for the Rushed by Sandi Richard
The Tin Fish Gourmet by Barbara-Jo McIntosh

Surfing

Canadian Living: Recipes
http://canadianliving.com/CanadianLiving/client/en/
Food/ListRecipe.asp?IdSM=379
Chatelaine: Food & Recipes
http://www.chatelaine.com/foodrecipes/
index.jsp?nID=8&pID=24
Cooking for the Rushed
http://www.cookingfortherushed.com
Epicurious
http://www.epicurious.com

171

Mayo Clinic: Healthy Recipes

http://www.mayoclinic.com/health/healthy-recipes/
RE99999

Meal Makeover Moms

http://www.mealmakeovermoms.com/recipes/index.html

Organized Home: Freezer Cooking

http://www.organizedhome.com/content-85.html

Real Simple: Recipes

http://www.realsimple.com/realsimple/channel/meal

Today's Parent: Food & Nutrition

http://www.todaysparent.com/food/index.jsp

APPENDIX D: MORE INFORMATION ON ALLERGIES

American Academy of Allergy, Asthma, and Immunology
   http://www.aaaai.org
Canadian Allergy, Asthma, and Immunology Foundation
   http://www.allergyfoundation.ca
The Food Allergy & Anaphylaxis Network
   http://www.foodallergy.org
Joneja Food Allergen Scale
   http://www.hallpublications.com/title2_sample1.html
National Institute of Allergy and Infectious Diseases
   www3.niaid.nih.gov

When it comes to health, information is always changing and being updated, so reliable online sources are often the most relevant resources to search for the answers to your questions.

Surfing

American Academy of Pediatrics

    http://www.aap.org/

BabyCenter

    http://www.babycenter.com/ *This is one of the largest commercial pregnancy and parenting websites. Features parenting articles, message boards, and other online resources that you'll want to know about at this stage in your parenting career.*

Canadian Health Network

    http://www.canadian-health-network.ca/

Canadian Paediatric Society
    http://www.cps.ca/
Caring for Kids
    http://www.caringforkids.cps.ca/ *Child health information
    for parents from the Canadian Paediatric Society*
Environmental Working Group: Wallet Guide to Pesticides
    in Produce
    http://www.ewg.org/sites/foodnews/walletguide.php
Health Canada
    http://www.hc-sc.gc.ca/
Women's Health Matters
    http://www.womenshealthmatters.ca/
Zero to Three
    http://www.zerotothree.org/

INDEX

178

healthy mum, happy baby

RECIPE INDEX

recipe index